FIGHT LIKE A GIRL

AN EMPOWERING SELF-DEFENCE
GUIDE FOR ALL WOMEN

FIGHT LIKE A GIRL

DELLA O'SULLIVAN

HarperCollins*Publishers*

HarperCollins*Publishers*
1 London Bridge Street
London SE1 9GF

www.harpercollins.co.uk

HarperCollins*Publishers*
Macken House, 39/40 Mayor Street Upper
Dublin 1, D01 C9W8, Ireland

First published by HarperCollins*Publishers* 2023

1 3 5 7 9 10 8 6 4 2

Text © Della O'Sullivan 2023
Illustrations © Becky Glass 2023

Della O'Sullivan asserts the moral right to be identified as the author of
this work

A catalogue record of this book is available from the British Library

ISBN 978-0-00-854679-3

Printed and bound in the UK using 100% renewable electricity at CPI
Group (UK) Ltd

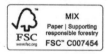

This book is produced from independently certified FSC™ paper to
ensure responsible forest management.

For more information visit: www.harpercollins.co.uk/green

For my late mother, Helen,
who will forever be my light of love.

CONTENTS

NOTE FROM THE AUTHOR

There are an endless number of moves and techniques you can learn from taking a martial arts or self-defence course. This book focuses on the basic mentality you can develop from taking these courses, as well as outlining the essential and more intuitive moves you can use to defend yourself on a day-to-day basis. It is impossible to note down every single move in one book, but I hope that what is included will inspire you to seek further training and at the very least leave you feeling empowered.

INTRODUCTION

This book is tailored to women, girls and marginalised genders of all ages and abilities, but it is a guide for anyone and everyone who wants to learn.

It is a first step for those who are a complete novice in self-defence or may have thought about taking a course and want a bit of insight. Maybe you have already begun training or maybe you just want to know how to handle yourself in different situations. Either way, you will find lots of useful information in these pages.

This book has two objectives: to empower its readers and to provide useful, adaptable knowledge. It is a condensed version of what I have learnt during my self-defence journey, which you can use as you see fit. It can be referred to if you decide to take up training or if you don't. It may just be the difference between having some knowledge to work with rather than none.

Women have always been considered the weaker sex, particularly in the physical sense, so the approach here is crucial. Together we will look at the best ways to approach self-defence as a woman, but this information is useful to all genders. To fight like a girl, you don't need to have 15 years of training. You don't need to imitate another person or gender. If you can learn skills that do not depend on your own physical strength and instead borrow the strength of an opponent, you will always have more time and energy at your disposal when you need it most.

But it's not just about self-defence in the physical sense.

It is fair to say that most people who learn self-defence do so either because they want to have the skills to protect themselves if they are faced with violence one day, or because they have already faced it and never want it to happen again. It's also fair to say that violence towards women and marginalised genders is disproportionately high, so many people learn self-defence because they think violence against them is not only possible, but likely.

The statistics bear this out. Globally, an estimated 736 million women – almost one in three – have been subjected to physical and/or sexual intimate-partner violence, non-partner sexual violence or both at least once in their life (that's 30 per cent of women aged 15 and older).[1] And in the last 12 months, one in five people in the LGBTQ+ community have experienced hate crimes, violence and domestic abuse.[2]

However, it's very important when learning these skills that we do so through a lens that will empower and not frighten, that we are not running on fear or high alert, but instead appropriating fear to help us be present and aware. I know from my own experience as a survivor that this mindset shift makes a big difference not only to how we feel, but also to our ability to defend ourselves effectively. Self-defence consists of physical skills, of course, but also mental skills – particularly inner strength and self-worth.

I learned the physical skills I possess from training, but I discovered how important it is to appropriate fear rather than run on it through my own research, introspection, therapy and personal growth.

When I reached a good standard in my self-defence skills my sense of awareness was heightened, but it wasn't a positive awareness; it was like being on high alert all the time, which is not a healthy state to be in. It just doesn't feel empowering or good, but it is there for a lot of us because of the disproportionate amount of violence women experience. I later learned that this is a common response to trauma in survivors, and unfortunately it doesn't disappear when you know only how to defend yourself physically. Marrying physical defence skills with the right mentality is vital to stop us running on fear, because being fully empowered is about feeling centred, present and physically strong all together.

I will take you through every stage necessary for self-empowerment through self-defence – including mentality, self-belief, the importance of setting boundaries (both physical and emotional), how to spot and assess a threat, what to do if there is a threat and how to be aware and present.

I will also cover how to remain composed under pressure, how to spot relationship red flags, how to overcome freezing (being in an immobilised state when faced with danger) and what happens when we experience the 'fight or flight' response. Each section will cover a specific topic to open your eyes to what you could potentially do with the right information but will present it in a way that will enable you to remember and utilise the information, as well as adapt it in all walks of life.

These are life skills, not just life-saving skills.

....

When I was asked to write this book, I thought a lot about how I would do that – how I can help those who want to learn through a book and what that would look like. I felt an introduction to self-defence with examples of the most common scenarios, techniques and topics was the best method, because it can always be referred back to. It can also be used with any practical style of self-defence. I also thought about what the book would represent and how to align that with the correct approach as a martial artist, as a woman and as a survivor.

Some women (like me) take up self-defence because they are survivors. They know what it feels like to have no one come to their aid, to feel utterly alone, and they use self-defence as a way to take back that power and build their self-confidence. Trauma of this kind doesn't go away once the violence stops. Survivors spend years picking up the pieces and regaining the self-worth that was stolen from them.

So, from the outset I would like to make my readers very aware of my stance when it comes to tackling the issue of male violence. *Fight Like a Girl* is *not* about changing your behaviour so that perpetrators don't have to change theirs. It is *not* being presented as a solution to what is a systemic and societal issue. In fact, anything we choose to do or not do – what we wear, whether we walk, run, don't run, smile, don't smile or just exist – has no place in the conversation when it comes to solving this problem. The issue is not ours to solve. It's not our responsibility. The onus is, and *solely* should be, on the *perpetrators*.

When women's self-defence is presented as a way to *solve* this issue, particularly by the people who have the power to address it on a systemic, structural and societal level, it derails the conversation. I wholeheartedly believe that we shouldn't have to learn self-defence to be safe. But having an interest in learning is okay too, and that interest should be your prerogative. It should be there to empower you, not to change or prevent a very real issue, because it is not your duty to do that. It is also not a go-ahead for others to use what you do as an example of what all women should do.

For me, this feels liberating: that, if needed, I can show up for myself and simultaneously agree that yes, I don't *need* saving, but that doesn't mean I don't *deserve* the basic human right to be and feel safe when walking down the street or to have the issues that impact my safety be addressed. One doesn't, nor should it, rule out the other.

I am not part of the victim-blaming party. I find it extremely offensive when people try to use what I have done as an example to other women, as if to say, 'See, if you just did this, problem solved.' I would like to live in a world where I am not likely to need to pull out my symbolic sword every time I leave the house. The fact that I have one is irrelevant.

When I explain to others why it's not okay for the powers that be to present self-defence as a primary solution when women express that they feel frightened, I use the swimming analogy. Learning to swim is great. It feels good and if you do fall in the water, you don't drown. But if learning to swim was presented to us as a solution to the rising waters caused by global warming instead of tackling the actual cause, people would think it ridiculous and an insult to their intelligence. Well, that's how most women feel when we are told to flag down a bus if we fear a policeman will harm us, or to take up self-defence and the problem is solved. The issue is huge – it is not a small swimming pool here and there that we may come across; it's a tidal wave.

I shouldn't have had to, but after I experienced on far too many occasions that my 'no' meant nothing, I decided to learn how to defend myself – this was my prerogative, not my duty. It should have been something I learned because it had been an interest of mine from the moment I saw Bruce Lee on my TV screen, not because I was scared for my life. And although the world is changing and conversations are starting to be had, things aren't changing fast enough.

Using self-defence is always a last resort – what I call having 'a last arrow' – but for many of us it feels like the only arrow we have, which is why there's a surge of women calling to book lessons every time there's a news report of yet another act of violence against women. It's the same reason I invite local MPs and councillors to attend my workshops – because they are full of voices that need to be heard.

I would like to see the martial arts have more spaces dedicated to women, and to see them more often taken up by women for the same reasons they take up dance or yoga – because it makes them feel empowered, because it brings balance to their lives or simply because they *enjoy* it.

Although my reason for taking up martial arts was quite negative, my reason for staying wasn't. I saw the real value of the discipline beyond my ability to throw hands. In the words of Joan Didion, 'I … lost touch with a couple of people I used to be',[3] but martial arts allowed me to see that just because I couldn't defend myself once, because I was fearful once, that didn't mean I would be defenceless and fearful in the future. Over time, I started to shed all the sticky feelings of shame and the sense of broken self-worth that my experiences had left me with. I rediscovered my forgotten self, who was hidden in the shadows of my trauma …

My experiences gave me the insight to know how important the correct approach to self-defence is, and it is why I have written this book through a lens that seeks liberation from the patriarchy. For longer than we can remember we women have been conditioned to believe we can't do certain things, that we are too small, too fragile … that we must be saved by good men. We have been taught that fighting is not for us, because global stereotypes have told society that we are terrible at most things, and that if we want to learn something physical, we have to become bigger, stronger, more aggressive. Then we might possibly be good at it … but only *for a girl* …

'You throw like a girl.'

'You run like a girl.'

'You're such a girl.'

'You fight like a girl.'

But, to me, fighting like a girl says I can be powerful in a way that doesn't require me to rely on strength; I can be powerful in ways that are natural to me; I have access to power too – it may not look the same as your power, but it's there and I can claim it.

I wanted to reclaim the insult 'like a girl' and turn it into something badass, because it is! In fact, Wing Tsun, the main art I studied, was founded by a woman and named after a girl who was her first student, so you will literally learn how to fight like a girl. And in a sense we already do, all day, every day. We overcome such heavy things, it's a wonder that 'like a girl' was ever accepted as an insult. I hope that if you ever hear that line said in a derogatory manner again after reading this book, you can say back, 'Yeah … I bloody well do.'

This book is inspired by every single woman and girl I have taught and met through my Fight Like a Girl classes and workshops over the years. A vast majority of them have been exposed to violence and abuse and have had to work through very real traumas. For some it took six or seven attempts to feel confident enough just to book a place. Their bravery astounds me.

This book also includes my own personal experiences as a survivor, and my journey through that, but this is married with my extensive knowledge and understanding of self-protection and martial arts, and indeed 'fighting like a girl'. (I am very small, and most of my training partners have been big men.) I have dedicated my life to mastery of this discipline. I have tested it and been tested on it, and now I feel I am one of the foremost experts in my field. Because I know exactly what it is like to feel frozen in fear and then have to find a way to overcome that. I know what our greatest attributes can be, and what kind of challenges we are likely to face when it comes to self-protection.

This book is me passing on the torch – one I wish I'd been handed some 20 years ago.

1.

MY STORY

I am from Peckham, South-east London.

My dad is a self-educated socialist. He taught me that you can never know enough; to always be a seeker of knowledge. My mother was a Cypriot woman who stood even smaller than me but was a true beacon of light. She was the best mother: honest, kind, nurturing and fierce.

I grew up on the same council estate as my grandparents and many of my cousins. Yaya and Bapu (my grandparents) looked after us kids many times – a house full of my 25-plus cousins. They were a major influence in my upbringing and contributed to my core values.

Our family motto was 'Never give up and never give in' – a slogan that later saved my life.

As a child, I did many activities, including gymnastics and dance, and always played well with other kids. I didn't lack confidence but have always been an introverted extrovert.

In my adolescence I crossed paths with an individual who went on to harass, stalk and physically assault me on numerous occasions over time. I didn't realise the full gravity of my situation until I became a mother, and particularly when I started learning more about psychology. I read about the red flags that identify very dangerous individuals, and about the countless other women whose stalkers went on to do them serious harm. These case studies really brought home to me the danger I was in, as they described the very same patterns of behaviour, language and situations I was experiencing.

The harassment began when I tried to set a boundary after he behaved in a way that was not okay with me. His reaction was terrifying and from that moment on, once that mask had slipped, I was thrown into a world I once thought I would never escape.

Threatening calls and texts were a daily occurrence, as was him turning up unannounced in places I was known to be. I did call the police on a few occasions, but at the time stalking was not considered a crime on its own, and I was told that this was all probably *just* to try to scare me. I was left feeling let down, like I was exaggerating or wasting police time, so even when things did escalate I didn't call them again.

Like many survivors, I felt shame, and because of that I hid most of what was happening from my family, although they knew about some of it. They didn't know the worst things, though, and this was because I feared for their safety and that their reaction might make things even worse. True or not, that's what I felt, because that's what I'd been told would happen by my abuser, and I was only a teenager.

Through all these public encounters only two people helped me: one was a cab driver who pulled up next to me and told me to jump in his cab; the other was a woman who actually walked right up to me and told me to get in her car, and with total conviction she said something to him that made him pause and back off. I can't remember what it was, but her presence shifted things and gave me an escape.

That amazing, brave lady demonstrated a power that still inspires me now, and I will never forget her.

There were so many other incidents – too many to list – but a handful have really stayed with me. They weren't always physical confrontations, but they were all terrifying, and the harassment felt relentless. As a result, I became a shadow of former myself and a ball of extreme anxiety all the time. Sometimes that would result in me acting out, and other times in me becoming a complete recluse. I stopped attending school regularly in Year 11 and my grades slipped. I didn't even turn up to one of my exams.

I was labelled as a troubled teenager by my educators. No one knew or bothered to look deeper.

These experiences sent me into a spiral and took over my life. I felt embarrassed, weak and stupid, so I just kept it all in or made out I wasn't feeling as terrible as I was inside. I even normalised this man's behaviours.

Eventually, for various reasons, his interest in me fizzled out and I managed to get away, but I continued to avoid going to certain places, and I just wanted to be with people all the time. I became co-dependent, which in turn suffocated my relationships. That uneasy feeling of looking over my shoulder was there all the time, and it was most intense when I was alone.

When I became a single mother, I began to have panic attacks at night. I was afraid of being alone in my flat with my baby boy. I started to have more frequent nightmares and flashbacks while I was awake – hearing a certain song, even queuing for a train, could trigger them. It became apparent that the fear I had felt was still in full force. I ended up making a lot of excuses to stay at my parents' house just so I could sleep at night.

Eventually I reached a point where I decided enough was enough. I was in a constant state of survival and operating fully on fear. I had no faith in myself. I was sick of looking for someone to come along to make me feel better, to save me. So I decided to stay on my own for a while and take up some healthy hobbies.

My brother introduced me to martial arts and brought me along for a trial lesson in a club. We'd grown up watching kung-fu movies, and I was always a fan of Bruce Lee and Jackie Chan. But I learned that this martial art I had been introduced to was what Bruce Lee had originally learned, and it had an even more impressive legend attached to it. The legend was that over 300 years ago this style was founded by a female kung-fu master called Ng Mui, and in her later years she trained a young woman called Yim Wing Chun, who sought out Ng Mui to teach her how to protect herself because she was being harassed and forced into marriage by the village bully.

That young woman was said to challenge this man after some years of training with the female master, and the challenge was that if she beat him in a fight, he would leave her alone. And it is said that she did just that.

Her chosen husband later learned this art from her, and he named the art in her honour.

As you can imagine that story was so inspiring for me at that stage in my life; I felt I could really relate to it. I wanted to be like Yim Wing Chun, and then one day be able to help other women, like Ng Mui. I felt so motivated. I thought, *This is it! This will help me overcome the fear I've been harbouring*, and because my brother was already training it didn't feel so scary to me to start training too.

However, it wasn't long before the triggers came, particularly when I was learning how to defend myself against certain attacks I had experienced in real time. But there were some great male training partners who had the best approach and made my training easier. They never knew how I was feeling or what I had experienced; they were just kind and patient. My training partner, Rob, was amazing. We went through all our grades together and, without knowing it, he really helped me.

Despite the triggers, I fell in love with it all. I trained every single day, and I never gave up on it or gave in to my fears. On days when I didn't feel motivated, I tapped into the discipline I'd learnt through martial arts to train regardless.

I developed fast, and got pretty good, but two years in I realised the training wasn't enough and that I should also start therapy. I began to work through a lot of the trauma with an amazing therapist, but for ten years I still told no one within my new world about my past and my reason for training.

I had imagined that by the time I attended my first master exam in 2016 I would be able to let go of the past and feel as powerful on the inside as I did on the outside. But I was still holding shame. Even then, I was a little shaky inside, and I believe this was because I still held the view that if all the people I taught, trained with and learned from knew that I was once a 'victim', they would look at me differently, negatively, and I would somehow lose their respect – and my own.

Then I was contacted by the *Evening Standard* and interviewed by a lovely reporter about my up-and-coming master exam. She loved that I, a small female, was going for a master grade within martial arts. As we spoke about my journey, she asked what had inspired me to train. I told her this and that, but I left out the real reason. After I hung up the phone, I instantly called her back – I literally did it so fast I couldn't talk myself out of it; I felt like this was the time. I was done with the shame.

I told her that this was the first time I was speaking out about what was a very personal experience – I told her what happened, and that none of my students knew my history, only my family, close friends and my sifu (teacher), and he only knew a tiny bit of information.

Having let it out, I felt a massive weight lift off me. I'd finally said it out loud. And the reporter's response was so reassuring – she sounded inspired, and for the first time I felt like none of what happened to me was my fault.

The article was printed on page three of the *Evening Standard* and was followed by interviews on BBC London.

What happened then was unexpected. I was inundated with calls and messages from women all over – some reached out from India – all to basically say, 'Hey, me too.' They thanked me for sharing my story, and several of them asked if I would consider running a class for women only. I was left so inspired. So from that soon followed the birth of the Fight Like a Girl women's self-defence programme, which went on to be featured on *ITV News*, radio stations and several other media outlets, and led to this very book being written.

The first workshop was one of the best days of my career. I felt that everything I had been through meant something now and had turned into something powerful. I could connect with and help those women in such a beautiful way; we shared our experiences, many of us for the first time. We'd created a safe space.

I realised then how important this was and that it was a stepping-stone for women, particularly survivors, towards healing and empowerment, and I have been teaching Fight Like a Girl ever since. It's adapted for any age, any ability. I have changed my approach over the years, learned more, done some unlearning, read lots of books, tested lots of moves, and I am better for it as a result.

I owe so much to all those women who sent me those messages, because they taught me that I was never a victim, but a survivor. I had never even heard that term before.

I have since set up Phoenix Eye, an inclusive martial arts association. I wanted to create a space for women, as I did through Fight Like a Girl, but also an inclusive space for all, and a space where women can continue to train with everyone. I do not tolerate any behaviours or language that would make anyone feel inferior or unsafe.

The name 'Phoenix Eye' is commonly known as a strike using the knuckle of your finger, and it happens to be one of my favourite techniques from one of the most beautiful forms I've learned. But that is not why I named the association Phoenix Eye. I named it after the phoenix from Chinese mythology.

The Chinese phoenix is a revered bird just like the Western phoenix, but its legend is more about what it does while alive rather than its rebirth. Its presence is only seen by those who are moral leaders, and it sits at the gates of empires. If any leader was to become corrupt the phoenix would leave. That is why there are statues of the phoenix at many building gates in China.

There are five Confucius virtues that are connected to each part of the phoenix:

1. The head represents morals and wisdom – the Chinese character is (DE) 德
2. The wing represents justice, honesty, righteousness, consideration for others, reciprocity, altruism – the character is 義 (YI)
3. The back represents propriety, courtesy, good manners, etiquette – the character is 禮 (LI)
4. The chest represents benevolence, kind-heartedness and humanity – the character is 仁 (REN)
5. The abdomen represents trustworthiness and integrity – the character is 信 (XIN)

I wanted to base the running of the association on these kinds of ethics, and to only allow those with moral virtues the privilege of helping others by teaching. In my opinion, teachers are there to help, to guide and ultimately to serve. The respect they gain should be earned and not demanded, and they certainly shouldn't be exploiting their students' enthusiasm and passion for learning.

2.

MENTAL DISCERNMENT AND SELF-BELIEF

For Kerry, and all that you helped me discover

Self-belief and self-worth are crucial components to effective self-defence. I wish I had known this from the start instead of figuring it out the hard way. Even if you simply want to learn to defend yourself physically, if you lack mental clarity, self-belief or self-worth, you will not execute the physical side with conviction or efficiency. I know this because I went through it. Trust the process, be patient with this chapter and take your time.

COMPOSURE AND FOCUS UNDER PRESSURE

Psychologists talk about the 'competence/confidence' cycle. This theory suggests that the more competent you are at something, the more confidence you have, and the more confidence you have, the more competent you will become. So of course if you have trained at anything consistently (fighting sports, driving cars, skateboarding, yoga), dedicating hours to developing a skill, over time your confidence in that area will grow because you know you are competent.

According to this theory, even if you start with little to no confidence, taking action to start something leads to confidence, because greater competence fuels self-belief, and then motivates you to take even more action.

Under real threat, however, everything is quite different. To maintain competence and efficiency under extreme circumstances you need to work on your mental and internal strength. When both are in tune, you will be able to show up as your authentic self, and make the leap from believing you can do something to knowing you can.

Mental discernment and self-belief lead to composure and focus under pressure

It is important to know that even those who have trained for years don't always have this down when it comes to real, intense . There are people who train regularly, who invest their time in combative sports and feel physically confident in a training environment, who will still freeze up, lose composure or have their focus and confidence shaken on the street.

I was one of them, and if I drop the ball, I still could be …

I thought my experience and my training alone was enough. I was taught that panic and fear are just natural biochemical reactions to danger, that it was natural to feel fear when under pressure, but I must learn to overcome it – the first part is true, but I now know fear doesn't need to be supressed; we don't need to get to a stage where we don't feel it. We need to get to a place where we are not controlled by it. At the time, I didn't just feel fear and panic. I was running on it 24/7!

What I learned was that I had an elevated response to fear because of my trauma. I had PTSD.

I realise not everyone reading this book will be a survivor, but because I am a survivor it took a lot of effort for me to gain self-belief and mental discernment – I had to work from the bottom up, and this deep understanding will hopefully benefit anyone who wants to develop in this area, no matter what level they are at. I wrote this book to offer knowledge and options to all, so you can take on what is useful for *you*.

Self-confidence is something I will probably continue to work on all my life, but the good news is that it's not exhausting. Over time it just becomes more of an awareness of what's going on within yourself and learning how to access the tools to recentre yourself when needed. I still have wobbles, but I now know how to show up for myself when I need to and interrupt the fear.

I have heard all the advice you can imagine over the years – 'just think positive', 'just believe in yourself' – and although it is good to aim for positive thoughts and self-belief, saying that to someone who doesn't know how to get there is not helpful. It is easy to tell someone to be confident if you don't know what it's like to have completely lost all confidence; it's easy to say have a strong mind if you haven't experienced years of self-doubt, or mental and physical abuse.

To get anywhere you need a map – you need to find and know the destination and then choose a route for how to get there. In this chapter I will share my map with you.

If anyone reading this has any form of past trauma similar to mine, I encourage you to see it as a true kindness to yourself to seek therapeutic support. I have done a lot of physical and mental work on myself, but I would have gone round and round in circles if I hadn't connected with my therapist. There is no shame in seeking help on this journey; the shame is not yours. To be empowered we need to allow ourselves the space to heal.

FEAR

'It's a tragedy to tell yourself not to be afraid.'
ANON.

Fear is generated in the part of our brain called the amygdala, also known as the 'lizard part'. It detects danger and triggers fear so that we instinctively stay away from that danger. (You will learn more about this in Chapter 4: Fight/Flight/Freeze.)

There are four triggers that enhance fear:

- Uncertainty
- Attention
- Change
- Struggle

These four triggers are likely to occur in a situation where you may need to defend yourself, when you feel: **uncertainty** at what might happen; unwanted **attention** forced upon you, and you having to focus your **attention** on the situation; a **change** from being comfortable and relaxed to feeling threatened; the **struggle** of having to find a way to safety.

Fear is appropriate in this context – it will be present in any dangerous situation, and it is very natural to feel it. When people have a fearless demeanour what they are demonstrating is the ability to maintain focus and composure, along with drive and determination, despite the fear. The fear may feel less intense to those who can do that, or they may just have an instinctive reaction to become mobilised when in danger (fight mode), but fear is still likely to be there.

The presence of fear alerts you to danger and can keep you focused in that moment. If you fear *feeling* fear and what that may say about you and your strength, however, you can end up running on fear and being run by it. That's when it's difficult to see and think clearly, find solutions and remain composed under pressure. It's when fear can turn into panic, and the benefits are not accessible.

How to interrupt fear

I used to have a major fear of flying. Whenever I was about to get on a plane or the plane was experiencing turbulence, the panic would rush in and trigger thoughts of the plane crashing, what that would be like and all the things I would miss out on.

I did see my therapist, Kerry, to help me overcome this fear, and in fact I dedicate this chapter to her. She gave me some exercises that helped me interrupt my fear of flying, but they were transferable to other running fears too. I had a fear of public performance and public speaking as well, something I am now able to do regularly. Below is one useful strategy you can try when you feel the panic rising:

1. Start by counting down from five to zero, or from ten to zero if required. This will interrupt any fearful thoughts and divert attention. You can imagine you are walking down steps as you count. Visualise walking down to your anchor thought.
2. Focus on a thought that makes you feel calm and happy – this is your anchor thought.

My personal anchor thought was an imaginary place I would visit where I felt at peace and happy. If I was on a flight, I would imagine arriving in the country I was travelling to and walking on the beach or training with my partners at the seminar, or I would think about the things I planned to do on arrival with friends and family. Then, whenever a fearful thought popped into my head, I simply said, 'Delete', and then repeated the process if it got to that level again. I also used this tool before I went for gradings (the assessments in martial arts), when I had to do public speaking or public performances.

Another tip on how to interrupt fear, which I use regularly, is to ask yourself a set of three questions to bring you back to the present moment. If you feel a bit wobbly, a bit off centre, anxious or frightened ...

Ask yourself:

'Who am I?'
'Where am I?'
'What time is it?'

And then answer:

I am '[insert name]'
'I am here.'
'It is now.'

The tone is important; ask the question strongly and clearly, and answer in the same way. This can help you tune in with the *now*, and be conscious and present when things become stressful or chaotic, particularly if you find yourself going over and over something that has already happened that you have no control over. Observation is okay; worry and panic is not. This is a tool I actually learned from one of my favourite books, *Way of the Peaceful Warrior* by Dan Millman, which is a semi-autobiographical work about a gymnast called Dan. His coach and mentor used those questions to help centre him in a present state. I still read that book every few years, and I have used those tools ever since I picked it up.

This is all about how we can keep showing up for ourselves, and if you make a conscious effort to practise this with every difficulty and challenge you face, you will become very good at it and therefore more likely to be able to access your present self if a dangerous situation does arise. Eventually it will become habitual and intuitive. If you are present, everything else is far more manageable.

HOW TO CONNECT WITH YOUR FIGHTING SPIRIT

Your fighting spirit is a feeling, an instinct, an innate need to survive. Accessing it enables your capacity to do whatever is necessary to be safe and can get you into a mobilised state, which is your fight or flight mode.

Using visualisation to find your fighting spirit

Visualisation is a powerful tool. Many athletes employ it, most famously the boxer Muhammad Ali, who routinely used affirmation, visualisation, mental rehearsal and self-confirmation to enhance his performance. This is said to be one of the reasons he would frequently say the words 'I am the greatest', to affirm that belief, as that is what he visualised himself being.

I have had many uncomfortable conversations where I knew the person would try to change my mind or twist, lie, plead, manipulate or make me feel like I was imagining things. When mentally preparing myself for these conversations I naturally felt anxious, so I rehearsed the conversation, I visualised showing up for myself and managing it well, and as a result I was as sharp as a sword in everything I needed to say. I did not lose composure or control. Visualisation was key for me to achieve what I wanted from the situation.

The power of visualisation has been backed up by various studies. In *Psychology Today*, it was reported that 'thoughts produce the same mental instructions as actions. Mental imagery impacts many cognitive processes in the brain, so the brain is getting trained for actual performance during visualisation. It's been found that mental practices can enhance motivation, increase confidence and self-efficiency, and prime your brain for success and increase states of flow.'[4]

So, I invite you to think of a time when you did something despite being scared or even just nervous, a time when you showed up as your authentic self, when you didn't need to push or pull or fight for what you wanted; you either just said it or did it. Connect that vision with your heart's centre, remember that feeling of being, speaking, walking and breathing, and keep visiting that memory. Allow the feeling of that memory to be present when you are training or visualising defending yourself.

If you are comfortable where you are now and in a safe space and you do have a memory of when you managed a really difficult situation well, check in with that now. Think of that time when you felt scared but you took action anyway, when you reacted instinctively and not because there was nothing to be afraid of. It could be any kind of situation that arouses those thoughts and feelings.

If you can't access that memory or don't have memories like this, that's okay, just think of a time when you showed up for someone else. And if that is not possible, you can simply *borrow* the experience of others. Look up the amazing survival stories of people who did what they needed to do, people you can relate to, like someone rushing to pull someone out of a burning building. Watch great scenes of communication like Julia Roberts in *Erin Brockovich* and see how she managed situations with conviction that everyone else thought were beyond her. Sometimes we need an 'ideal', an inspiration or an icon to guide our visualisations.

Alternatively, you can picture a scenario of what it would take to get you to react or do something even if you were scared. Ask yourself how you would want to manage a situation like that and visualise!

I'll introduce you to one of mine:

The lioness

Why is she great? Because she is the iconic mother. She harbours unconditional love – and what's that going to do? It makes her a force to be reckoned with. She is a knowing mother, non-judgemental and present. She has implicit knowledge, and she is revered by the male lions.

I am a mother myself, and at the beginning of my training this was all I had to tap into. I lacked the motivation and confidence when I thought about protecting myself, but as a mother I have an innate impulse to protect, and I will do so fiercely. So when I thought about what I would do if I needed to protect my little boy, there was the lioness. And I felt my body language adjust and my mind shift. Physiological and psychological changes were happening; I even felt my pupils dilate. I could connect with my fighting spirit; even though at the time it was small, I gained confidence from knowing it was there. I just needed to grow it. This is a tool that I encourage you to try to use if you feel you would not respond in the best way if it were just yourself you were showing up for. Show up for someone else. Visualise being the lioness.

This is not to encourage you to want to rip someone's face off if they cross you; it's a way for you to access the capacity to defend yourself when needed and connect with that feeling through visualisation, particularly if you feel you are prone to freezing. People who can access this naturally may not need to do this – however, I wasn't one of them.

If you can connect with that fighting spirit and draw it in, the good news is that you know it is there, it exists! Now you can use this to show up for yourself as well as for other people.

We have to allow ourselves this same motivation and instinctive response to protect our own lives. In my own journey, I was left pondering why I struggled so much when it came to thinking about showing up for myself.

The main reasons that came up were:

- Lack of self-worth
- Lack of self-belief
- Past traumas
- No self-confidence

Which all resulted in my nervous system being out of whack. It may be the same for you, it may be different, or you may not have trouble in this area at all. Either way, we are making a map towards empowerment, and our thoughts have the power to shape that journey. When using visualisation as a tool to access your fighting spirit, keep these points in mind:

- Changing our thoughts changes our beliefs.
- What we think effects how we feel.
- If we think and feel something enough it changes our belief system and then we operate in the world within that belief system.

Just because you couldn't or didn't show up for yourself once doesn't mean you cannot in the future, which is why shifting those thought patterns is vital.

ACCEPTANCE: THE ART OF CONTROLLING THINGS

If you only focus on the problem, you will never find the solution.
KUNG-FU PRINCIPLE

Life is full of situations that shouldn't be the way they are. Sometimes you can fix these situations, but sometimes you can't. Accepting things as they are is a powerful way to cope with what is out of your control.

If you can accept what you *cannot* control, you can shift your focus to what you can control and what *is* available to you, and you will be all the more empowered for it. When I say accept, I do not mean to accept defeat. If you spend your time constantly trying to fight what you have no power over you will waste your time and energy, and you will still be left with the problem.

There are times when you should hold yourself accountable, but you should never blame yourself for things you have no control over. There is a difference between falling into a situation because you do not know better or have been manipulated and choosing to be in a situation because of your ego. Take these two examples below:

Situation 1: You've been dating someone for a few months, and they accuse you of flirting with another person and use that as an excuse to justify their abuse, whether physical or mental. This is not a situation where you are to blame. It is the perpetrator who is accountable.

Situation 2: You're at a club with your friends and someone bumps into you. Rather than ignoring the action, you react negatively and shove them back, initiating a fight. In this situation, you are as much at fault as the other person and you should be held accountable.

Accepting what you cannot control will allow you to spot the possible courses of action that can actually help you.

How to use acceptance in a non-threatening scenario: You have lost your job, and you feel crappy about it. You cannot change that you have lost your job, and you also cannot change that it doesn't feel great. Trying to suppress these emotions is just as bad as trying to beg your boss for your job back. But being consumed by them can lead to unhelpful and inaccurate thoughts about yourself and can blind you to the solution.

Instead, allow yourself to feel whatever you are feeling and don't punish yourself for it. Be kind to yourself: express and process how you feel. You can journal, you can speak to a friend, but give yourself the space to *witness* your emotions; they will pass more naturally, and you will be better able to find a solution. If you suppress your emotions and swim against the current, the next time something similar happens, that current will be a tidal wave.

How to use the art of acceptance in a self-defence scenario: Someone grabs your wrist really tightly and pulls you towards them. You naturally feel extremely uncomfortable with this. You know you want them away from you and for their hand to no longer be on your wrist. But if you put all your focus on what you can't control (their hand around your wrist, because it's already happened, and they may be a lot stronger than you), you won't notice that your other hand is free. We tend to forget what's available to us when we focus on the problem. This is a classic example – most will try to pull in the opposite direction against a greater force, and completely forget that their other hand and legs can be used too.

Three reasons why it is good to accept things as they are

1. Trying to change what you have no control over can lead to feelings of bitterness, anger and sadness.
2. Acceptance allows you to recognise and face the actual problem.
3. Accepting things as they are leads us towards a sense of peace and calm, as if a burden has been removed.

How to accept things as they are

1. Notice when you are trying to change or deny things that can't be changed. For some people, warning signs include thoughts such as, *This is unfair! It shouldn't be this way!* Or, *Why me?* For others, the signs tend to be emotions such as anger or frustration.
2. Remind yourself that 'it is what it is'. If there is nothing you can do to change it right now, then to keep your head above water you must swim with the current. You may need to do this multiple times a day, depending on the situation.
3. Allow yourself to feel sad and disappointed; these feelings are healthy! At the same time, trust that acceptance will eventually bring you peace and calm.
4. Seek out social support. Engage in self-care activities to help you cope and improve your mood. See it as a gift to yourself.

Now, when I am aware that I'm running on old thoughts and feelings, I use these tools above to recentre myself. But when I was still working on my internal dialogue I would often say things to myself like: 'This always happens to me …' 'What did I do to deserve this?' And the truth was, I didn't do anything to deserve any of the bad treatment in those situations, and how I was treated wasn't a reflection of me. What people choose to do and how people choose to treat others is a reflection of them. It rarely has anything to do with you.

'What we think about ourselves we tend to believe.'
UNKNOWN

Your internal dialogue has a direct impact on how you feel and what you think about yourself. Let's say you are about to go into a meeting or a conversation with someone who has a history of manipulative behaviour, who takes every boundary you set as a personal attack and is defensive. Maybe it's a boss who never listens and keeps finding ways of roping you into more work without more pay.

Before you go into the conversation you could say something empowering and reassuring to yourself, such as: 'I know how it feels to be aligned with what serves me.' Just that little statement can put you in a much better space to be clear and to set boundaries.

Find the positives in the negatives.
KUNG-FU PRINCIPLE

Once we can accept what we *cannot* control, we can see what we *can* control and find the advantages in a situation – even when the negatives are more obvious.

Below is an example of a negative situation, and two types of thought pattern that could result from it. Number one lays out the obvious negatives, and number two lays out the positives and things that are helpful to pay attention to.

Imagine that a man has come by and grabbed you by both your arms. The negatives are obvious:

1.

- He is stronger than me.
- He has hold of both my arms.
- He is very close, aggressive and scary.
- He might hit me.
- I can't move.

The positives may be less obvious, but they do exist:

2.

- He has tied up both of *his* hands.
- He has opened up all *his* vital targets (see Chapter 10: Controlling Attackers).
- I have the element of surprise.
- My hands, knees and elbows are still free.
- I am in close enough proximity to defend myself, so his longer range doesn't matter.

The second list of observations is far more helpful, because it involves what you can do and control; it shifts the focus from them to you. This is not ignoring what they are doing, but rather viewing all of what they are doing and how to use what they have done to your advantage.

SELF-WORTH AND SELF-DEFENCE

Our sense of self-worth has a direct impact on our mentality and confidence: if you do not see your value, this belief will impact on your ability to come to your own aid. This is why abusers aim to diminish a person's self-worth. They break you down bit by bit, to the point where you are easily controlled and will find it so much harder to find a way out.

This is how abuse works, and why it's so damaging to say things such as 'Why didn't you just leave?' to someone who has survived violence or is still in an abusive relationship.

It is not just getting away that gives you your life back, it's picking up the pieces afterwards and trying to find that forgotten self you once knew – that girl who used to walk with her head held high, with confidence in her eyes and fire in her belly.

I know that feeling. I had to search for my forgotten self too, and sometimes I still do.

If you don't believe you are enough, you can feel already defeated internally. To shift this, a helpful and healthy internal dialogue needs to happen.

Introspection

Introspection is inner work. It improves self-awareness and leaves you more conscious of your thoughts and feelings. It is tapping into your mental state, and trying to identify any patterns, what you believe about yourself, what you tell yourself, and how those thoughts and feelings affect your behaviours.

If you want to have a strong mental state, you need to have self-confidence, and to have confidence in an area you need to understand it well.

To understand others, we must first understand ourselves.
KUNG-FU PRINCIPLE

In my discipline, this philosophical lesson is for the first stage of learning when you are practising defence against one average attacker. At every stage there is internal work tied to it, but this first stage is a form of introspection: to build confidence by understanding yourself. Below are some introspective exercises to help you do just that:

- Name how you're feeling at any given moment.
- Understand your emotional triggers.
- List your strengths and shortcomings in context.
- Recognise your impact on your surroundings.
- Make decisions with intention and purpose.
- Observe your interactions: do you keep eye contact? Do you interrupt people or give them time to speak?
- Use positive language and affirmations – 'I am worthy.' 'I am kind.' 'I do not need to people-please to know that I am kind.'

If you find yourself seeking validation through others, start making a conscious decision to do something for yourself and keep it to yourself, even if it's as simple as setting a boundary for your alone time, like having a bubble bath with no disturbances. Doing things to seek validation from others doesn't help with self-confidence; it's great to be kind, and to do kind things because you like being kind, but if you do them because you think that's how you can feel validated or worthy, this is not being kind to yourself.

Seek the bridge

The next stage in building self-confidence, which I learned after introspection, was to 'seek the bridge'. This means to bridge to others: observe how you interact with others, and how you see things from other people's perspective. In a self-defence context this means trying to read your opponent, recognising behavioural red flags and assessing their intent.

Stop playing the wrong movies

Playing the wrong movie basically means replaying something that was not your fault in your head and assigning the blame to yourself. I was doing this quite often, and my therapist Kerry brought this to my attention, calling me out on the fact that I was misremembering how certain scenes actually played out.

I was doing this because I was trying to understand why I was mistreated. I did so by putting myself in their shoes, and I thought, *Gosh, I would have to really hate someone to treat them that way*. My rationalising was telling me that those people must hate me, and that thought really hurt me, because I was kind to them. I didn't deserve any hate, and I already had low self-worth. At the time I put so much value on what others thought of me. I told myself that as this keeps happening, it must be because of me; it was a flaw in *my* character.

I am the common denominator here.

This is a common thought pattern when we are shocked by how someone treats us. For me, it was my inability to understand another person's perspective. Putting myself in their shoes wasn't helpful, because I am not like them and I wouldn't do what they did. Seeing and accepting them for who they actually are based on their actions was more helpful. Kerry helped me see that their behaviour wasn't a reflection of *me*, it was a reflection of *them* and what's going on inside of them.

The shame I was holding onto from my days of abuse wasn't mine to hold. I started to see things differently. I didn't need to change who I was; I just needed to rediscover and value myself in order to protect myself from people who wanted to harm me. I could no longer ignore the red flags because of how I felt or the charming words they used. The greatest realisation was that I didn't need to become cold or cruel to do this. You can still be kind and good, and have a big heart, while being loyal to yourself. So whenever you are processing something, make sure to check in with your throughs and notice if you are replaying the 'wrong movie'.

TIP: If you want to change anything you believe about yourself, you can write it on a Post-it note and stick it around the house. Remember: what we tell ourselves we tend to believe ...

KNOWING YOUR BOUNDARIES

If you do not know what your boundaries are, and you do not get used to setting them in all areas of your life, I can tell you for a fact that this mentality will spill into your ability to effectively defend yourself. If you cannot set emotional boundaries and are not used to defending yourself on the most basic level, you will likely struggle to set boundaries with a person who poses a physical threat to you.

First, we have to establish what our boundaries look like and how to be loyal to ourselves when it comes to setting them.

What lives on your centre line?

Kung-fu principles often have dual meanings and they are normally both physical and philosophical. This is so you can develop the mentality, the internal growth and the physical skills all at the same time. The 'centre line' is one of those principles. In the physical sense, it refers to the central line of the body. The weakest targets on the human body are close to this line, so this is where it is best to position our hands when preparing to defend ourselves. It allows us to protect our own centre line, but also to have the shortest, most direct and most efficient line of attack to our opponents (see page 120 for more on defending and attacking from your centre line).

The philosophical meaning behind the centre line, however, is about knowing your boundaries. If you do not know what your boundaries are, you will find it difficult to set them, and in martial arts we call this knowing your line – this is your personal, emotional and spiritual 'centre line'; where you place value – the things that you are not willing to compromise on for anyone.

So what are your lines? What do you view as acceptable or unacceptable behaviour? It is important to pay attention to how you feel in your interactions with others (friends, colleagues, family, romantic interests). Is there anything that people have said or done that has made you feel uncomfortable? What are you happy to share with work colleagues and friends? What are your deal breakers? If someone has said or done something that is a deal breaker for you, you need to be prepared to access what I call 'an emotional samurai sword' and sever the ties with that person when the time comes.

Things that could live on your centre line

— Morals – not compromising them for others.
— Respect – not engaging in or continuing a conversation with those who lack respect.
— Self-control – removing yourself from a situation or conversation with someone who is being controlled by their emotions.
— Awareness – not ignoring red flags when you see them.
— Family – prioritising what's really important.
— Your body – it's your own, it doesn't belong to anyone else and no one else is entitled to it. Set the tone with what you are comfortable with when it comes to your body. This includes what you wear, and what you share.

Exercise

Now I want to invite you to take a moment to fill in your own personal list of what lives on your centre line. List the things that are most important to you, the people who are most important to you and the boundaries you want to set. I have put one of my own boundaries down as an example to start you off.

Ask yourself: **What is truly important to me?**

WHAT LIVES ON YOUR CENTRE LINE?	BOUNDARY
e.g. honesty	I will always strive to be a good communicator and I will accept people in my life who can respect my value of honesty.

Once you've done this, take a look at the positive statements below, which will help to reinforce your loyalty to yourself and your boundaries:

- I know how to live in line with my priorities and my boundaries.
- I know how it feels to have clear boundaries that are best for me.
- I know how to communicate my needs and boundaries effectively.

THE BEST VERSION OF YOURSELF

Just as you might use an ideal or icon to inspire your fighting spirit, you can also use one to inspire your internal strength., so here I want to introduce another muse: the best version of yourself.

This version of yourself is at the very least your forgotten self, and at the very best your forgotten but rediscovered self. At the very centre of this figure is all of you – past, present and future, with all of your flaws accepted – though that doesn't mean being stagnant; you are still ever changing, ever moving, and you should always aim to keep growing. You can use other inspirations when needed, of course, but it is such a powerful thing to be able to connect with and be inspired by yourself.

The only way you can truly show up for yourself in this way is if you have self-acceptance and self-love, and really start to like yourself and look out for yourself as you would a best friend or family member. Think about what the best version of yourself looks like, picture that person and see them doing all the things you ever wanted to do and really living, feeling grounded, present, aware and happy! And when you feel low, have that version turn up for you.

Whenever you feel alone, show up for yourself.
DELLA O'SULLIVAN

3.

AWARENESS AND PLANNING

'Being aware is being present, and being present
gifts you with foresight.'
DELLA O'SULLIVAN

Being aware is not the same as being on high alert. When you are aware, you know when to be more vigilant, alert and focused. Awareness should make you feel more grounded and present. It stops you from being easily distracted, from rushing or stumbling. It will allow you to be calm even in times of chaos.

INTUITION

It's important to remember that sometimes you can be hyper-vigilant and aware, and do everything imaginable to prevent or protect yourself, but some people are just tricky, convincing or very good at hiding in the shadows. Your intuition is a very real thing. If you feel something is off, if your intuition is flaring up, listen to it. It is often our subconscious picking up on something our conscious mind has missed. Awareness of your own intuition is part of the journey.

Gut feelings you should not ignore

- An uncomfortable feeling someone has given you. There have been so many cases where it comes to light that a person who has committed horrible crimes left others they've met feeling uncomfortable, despite not knowing anything about them or their activities. If you feel that, tune into it and pay attention!
- Unwanted touching and attention – when someone is always making an excuse to be physical with you. They may make a joke of it or make it seem like they are doing something nice for you, even though you've made your boundaries clear. This is to minimise your reaction or prompt you not to be too firm. If you feel uncomfortable, trust that feeling.
- You see the same person more than once in more than one location, and it's not a good feeling when you do.

Listen to your instincts and know that if you feel uncomfortable, you can make your exit. This is not just about running away from a threat, but also knowing that it's okay to change your mind if you simply decide you want to remove yourself from a situation. For example, you might have planned a date with someone but it feels off and so you don't want to continue it, or you might feel the dynamic of a party isn't what you are comfortable with. Make sure you are not leaving a friend in danger and that your exit is safe first, but otherwise, wanting to leave is enough, even if it is based on gut feeling alone.

AWARENESS IS YOUR FRIEND

When I was an assistant teacher, training bodyguards, I learned a lot from the participants about awareness. I would say 95 per cent were ex-military, and they said that when an incident suddenly occurs something has probably been missed at least three steps back.

So how do we learn not to miss things, and how do we know if we are aware enough or not? Well …

Have you ever lost something and found that when you tried to retrace your steps you could easily remember what route you took, who you saw on the way, if anything was different and at what point you last used the item? If you could do this easily then that is good news – you clearly have good awareness – but what if you took the same journey and this time you were in a hurry or so distracted by your thoughts, your phone or a conversation that you took a different turn to usual, and maybe someone brushed past you and you didn't notice them taking your wallet out of your pocket?

Awareness allows you the foresight to notice things early, and it doesn't only come in useful in a self-defence context. It can include things like moving aside when you can see someone is about to bump into you, moving a friend who is about to walk into something or avoiding a road accident.

So let's break down this misconception that increasing your awareness is hard work, because it doesn't need to involve a massive change in your behaviour. We already learn awareness in other areas: when we are crossing the road, riding a bike or driving a car; we are taught to notice things so that we can see things coming and take evasive action if necessary. In those situations, we stop ourselves from being distracted by phones or conversations and we take a moment to slow down, check our surroundings or look in our mirrors. These things become habitual and second nature, so we don't even realise we are doing it.

It takes little to no effort to keep your head up and your eyes open. It's about being present, and when you are present you are not only more conscious, but also happier and less stressed. And if a dangerous situation were to arise, you would be much more likely to see it early and be better prepared.

The mind of a perpetrator

During my time as an assistant teacher for a bodyguards' training unit, they covered this subject because their job was to spot things before they happen and to better protect their clients.

During the training the instructor laid out three main things that a perpetrator looks out for when setting eyes on a target. I found this very useful and, from my experience, I also found it to be very true:

1. A lack of awareness – they can see you're distracted or your senses are dimmed.
2. Someone who in their eyes appears to be a victim – someone they think will not fight back and whom they can easily overpower.

3. An isolated location – they will look for a way to easily isolate their target, taking them to or moving in on them when they are in a badly lit area or somewhere with few people around, or both.

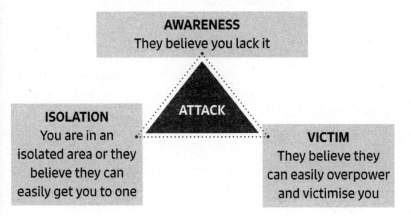

How *cowardly*, right?!

So now we have established what they look for, let's talk about how we can be more empowered by this knowledge, use it to our advantage and increase our chances of spotting shifty behaviour if it arises.

AWARENESS AND HOW TO INCREASE IT

Be present, be conscious – Start by making a conscious effort to notice when you are lost in thought. When this happens bring your attention to your breath and count five things you can see around you. This will help you be aware of your surroundings and keep your mind present. Just a small effort to check back in with where you are every so often will keep you aware. This is the reason meditation is such an important factor in martial arts and many other practices, because it teaches you to be present and alert.

Practise noticing things – Not only will this improve your memory and make you more aware, it will also help you know where to go in an emergency. I always ensure I do this, particularly when I am out with my girlfriends, my family and certainly my son when he was small. It allows me to know where to direct them in an emergency and where to go if we need help. It has also just made me enjoy my walks more – I enjoy my surroundings and stay aware at the same time, instead of being in my head.

Tips to increase awareness

Here's a checklist of things to notice, wherever you might be:

- Check the layout of the room you are in.
- Chose a seat that allows you to see the entire room.
- Look around the room of an establishment when you walk in.
- Take note of cameras, exits and how many people are at the bar.
- What time is it?
- What's the weather like outside?
- How many people are at the bus stop?
- How many security guards are at the door?

I am a huge fan of Sherlock Holmes, and I am studying criminal psychology, so to me this is an interesting and fun thing to do, particularly when I am alone. It is a very useful life skill to be observant – it can help you remember people and notice when someone might be upset or lost – so in your day-to-day life just practise taking a mental note of the people you meet; it could be the bus driver or the barista at the coffee shop. It's important to note, however, that you do not have to remember everything, as that can feel overwhelming. The idea is not to constantly scan the world looking for danger, but to develop a natural awareness, so that you notice things without feeling paranoid or fearful. With that in mind, think about the following:

— What's their general appearance?
— Height?
— Weight?
— Age?
— Hair colour?
— Markings (tattoos, scars, piercings)?
— Voice and accent?
— Smell?
— Anything else: do they walk a certain way, have an odd way of moving, were they holding anything, what were they wearing?

If you can practise doing this every so often and be more aware of the places and people around you, you will be more present and remember things about people. It's also helpful because remembering details about others is a good social skill.

Peripheral vision

We often ignore what we can see in our peripheral field of vision, but that could lead us to miss important information. A quick way to test your peripheral vision is by carrying out the following:

• Stand up and stretch your arms out in front of you and place your hands together.
• Slowly move each hand to either side of you at the same time.
• Stop when you can no longer see both hands.
• That is the marker for your peripheral vision.

To use your peripheral vision, practise looking towards something ahead of you and then also noticing other things around you. The key is:

a. Don't cover your peripheral vision with clothing, glasses, a phone, etc. (If you feel like you're in danger then remove these things.)

b. Focus on everything and nothing (i.e. don't focus your eyes on one thing ahead). Keep your head up and try to see everything, but don't focus on one thing.

Practise noticing things in your peripheral field. For example, I currently have my laptop in front of me (good job I can touch-type), with my phone to my left. My dog is sitting on the floor just to the right (very close to where the field ends); I have a book open to the right of me and I can still see my wardrobe on my right and my chest of drawers on the left. I can see the window in front of me and the details of my garden beyond that. Just taking note of these little things as I am doing something else has helped me develop an awareness of my surroundings.

Take your time

Have you ever been efficient at anything when in a rush? Have you ever made mistakes when you're in a rush? There is a reason for that. When we rush, we are flustered, we are distracted, and our awareness suffers.

Make it a rule that when you are travelling anywhere – to the car, to work, to the shopping centre, on the school run – you will not rush! And if you do have to hurry, ensure you do not compromise on your thinking time or your reaction (for example, speeding in a car). Rushing and panicking increase your chances of making mistakes, and that will make your journey or task longer, causing further panic and further problems.

Eyes

Keeping your eyes open and your vision unimpaired is essential for good awareness:

- Hoods and hats: If you want to put your hood up but still want to maintain your peripheral vision so you can see your surroundings, place the hood in line with or just behind your temple.
- Phones: We have all seen the videos of people online who are so glued to their phones that they end up walking into a fountain or lamppost. Phones are so useful, but they can draw us in and distract us terribly. Instead of hunching over your phone as you sit or walk, just lift your phone a little higher so that your head is almost straight. Just use your eyes to look at your phone rather than bending your neck, and make a conscious effort to look up regularly.

Ears

Our hearing is another vital sense when it comes to being aware of our surroundings:

- Earphones: Listen to your music, girl! But if you feel something isn't right and you do not feel safe, you can always turn your music down so that you can hear better, but other people don't know you can hear. This is sometimes useful when dealing with sexual harassment. It's easier to ignore the person when it appears that you cannot hear them. They won't know you can, and it keeps you alert if that person is drawing closer or becoming aggressive. Alternatively, you can always just have one earphone on. I always pull one earphone out when I am crossing the road, and if I am aware of someone present who I don't trust.

- Phones: Thieves will look for someone who is distracted by their phone. If you are out and about having a phone conversation, try using earphones, or put your phone on loudspeaker and hold it close to your mouth, on the physical centre line of your body (see page 119). Stay away from the edge of the pavement, as most moped phone thefts happen when someone is walking close to the edge of the pavement with their phone to their ear. The phone blocks their entire peripheral vision on one side, so they do not see the thief coming.

CONFIDENT BODY LANGUAGE AND VISUALLY ASSERTING YOURSELF

Do not change your behaviour so that someone else doesn't have to. I don't believe in this. I do, however, believe in human psychology, and that what we believe about ourselves manifests physically in our demeanour, in the way we sit, walk and communicate. And others will inevitably pick up on that.

For example, I know of a male martial artist who joined a club, trained really hard and became super-skilled because he was constantly getting bullied. However, because this man did not do any internal work (which he admitted himself) and gained no self-awareness through the process, his newfound aggression and confidence was so clear in his body language that it seemed to outsiders that he was challenging them to a fight. He may as well have been wearing a big red sign saying 'I dare you to fight me' – and people did try to fight him. He handled the situation well, which he was pleased about, but what he wasn't pleased about was that he had started this process to stop the unwanted attention, and now he was still getting it, just in a different way. Good for him, though, he had the humility to look at himself and adjust his body language.

The point here is that toughness doesn't always need to be on show; self-defence is the art of avoidance. I have met some of the most skilled people and you wouldn't even notice them in a room. They are both unassuming and present.

This is what we need to be. We don't need to look super-passive, because that attracts attention, and we don't need to be super-aggressive, because that also attracts attention. We just want to be ready and able, calm and present.

> *'What you feel will emit that energy.'*
> KERRY HOWARD, THERAPIST

Adjusting your body language is not for the benefit of others, it is for you, as the language we use, verbally or physically, affects what we think, feel and believe about ourselves. If you are interested to know what to do if someone wants to harm you physically, well, it all starts here in our thoughts. Notice when you are feeling defeated, low or sad, and try putting your shoulders back. Or, if you feel over-whelmed or frustrated, kneel on the floor, get grounded or even do some push-ups, as if you are literally pushing that feeling away from your heart's centre.

Empowering body language

As I suggested in Chapter 2: Mental Discernment and Self-belief, show up for yourself mentally first and you will find that your body language follows. This practice has aided me to feel grounded when anxiety has arisen. Try the following:

- When walking, create a posture you would imagine yourself having if you felt totally confident and knew your own worth. Keep that position. Now imagine a string pulling your head up towards the sky. Picture a straight line running from each earlobe through your shoulders, hips and ankles. This is a firm stance, which projects confidence both internally and externally. You will look tall no matter your height and it gives an energetic shift to how you may be feeling about yourself or if you feel worried about your walk home.

- When sitting, keep your back firmly against the back of your chair. Keep your feet planted on the ground; this will allow you to get up quickly without having to lean forwards.

- Even just the motion of swinging your arms a bit more than you normally would when you're walking can make you feel more confident, and the more confident you feel, the more confident you will look to others.

- Make eye contact – I know it can feel intimidating, but someone who avoids eye contact will appear distracted or lacking in confidence. And sometimes eye contact can teach you a lot about others' intentions. You do not have to make eye contact with someone you feel is a threat, just be aware of them, but in your day-to-day practices, when interacting with people, make an effort to make eye contact. A great tip is to imagine looking at the colour of someone's eyes instead of looking directly at their eyes. I find this less intimidating and a good way to maintain eye contact when I want to.

- Keep your chest up and your shoulders back always, even when sitting. Again, this demonstrates confidence and self-assurance. Try sitting with your shoulders curled forward and chest in, and see how that feels, then try putting your shoulders back and opening up your chest with you head pulled up and see how that feels. It really does make a difference to how we feel about ourselves *inside*.

ISOLATION AND LOCATION

'Let your intuition guide you.'
DELLA O'SULLIVAN

If it's late at night the darkness can hide many things that we can miss with the naked eye. Perpetrators often choose badly lit areas to hide in and launch their attacks from. Just ask yourself, would I feel comfortable walking this route with my child? Would I advise someone else to take this route? If the answer is no, give yourself that same kindness and avoid that route, **particularly if you feel something isn't right**.

If you feel you're at risk, always chose safety before all else.

Maybe someone has offered you a lift home and they are being persistent, but they make you feel uncomfortable or for whatever reason you don't trust them. Or maybe you are in a hurry to get home because you have been catcalled relentlessly on your way back on a Friday night, so you are thinking of taking the shortcut through the car park or park, or considering accepting that lift because that guy is being so persistent.

Remember: when someone doesn't respect your boundaries, it could be a red flag. So, ask yourself: does that person just want to ensure you get home safely or do you feel like they just want to be alone with you? If you are not comfortable with the answer then be firm and decline their offer. Know that it is okay to ask for help – it is not a weakness; there is strength in asking for it and accepting it.

Similarly, if you do feel unsafe at any point then put your safety above others' convenience. Peer pressure can and has directed all of us at some point to do things we do not want to do. Know your limits and that you can choose to say, 'I do not want another drink', if you feel uncomfortable, unwell, or that your faculties are impaired. Ask a friend you trust to drop you home instead of accepting the offer of someone you maybe don't know or are getting a bad gut feeling from. Call someone to collect you directly from a safe spot, especially if you keep seeing the same person in more than one location. Please show up for yourself in these situations as you would if you were witnessing a friend experiencing this.

Most of the things I list below I guarantee most women and people from marginalised communities already think about. These are things you can include in your habitual day-to-day practice – things I now do habitually without even thinking. If you do feel uneasy, threatened or harassed in some way, these precautions can help you be more prepared. Just a short note before we begin this section, though: it is not your responsibility to carry out these tasks. I have provided the information below as a guide to help increase your awareness, and because I've found it useful as someone who travels alone a lot, but you do not have to try to remember it all. I do not want anyone to feel overwhelmed here, so bear in mind that you will not be in all of these situations at the same time. Again, the idea is to give you empowerment through knowledge, not to incite fear and paranoia. And remember that, should something happen to you, it is not your fault. It is a societal issue that leads to people's lives being in danger. Doing the things listed below will not change society, and just because we *can* do these things, doesn't mean we *should have to*. These are simply actions you can take to allow yourself to feel safer and more at ease.

Badly lit streets

- Walk on the side of the street with the most houses.
- If you want to avoid a group of people, walk closer to the road.
- Walk in the road if it's super-quiet. If you find yourself on a street with a lot of parked cars, trees, walls and side alleys, walking down the centre of the road will give you time and space to move and not be easily isolated.

Blind spots

- Corners: When taking a corner walk widely around it so you can see who or what is coming from the other direction before you are physically there.
- Getting out of cars: Make a quick effort to check all mirrors before you exit, just as you would if you were to turn a corner or looking out for cyclists.
- Lifts: Position yourself so that your back is to the lift wall and not to people – I always choose a corner close to the exit so I can see all sides of the lift at once and get out quickly.

Quiet car parks

- If you can, park on high ground outside where you are easily seen by passers-by.
- If you have to use an underground car park, try to choose a space close to an exit, by a payment station and within sight of CCTV cameras.
- Reverse park so if you need to make a quick exit, you can do so easily.
- Before you leave your car check every mirror, and make sure you get out with your eyes on the road. Keep your hands as empty as possible.

Dark, secluded parks and paths

- Choose paths that are well lit.
- Choose the wider paths.
- Walk the path that has a café on it!

If you feel someone walking up behind you

- You can step to the side to let them pass or walk around a parked car so that an obstacle is between you and the person approaching you (more about this in Chapter 8: Strategies and Tactics). If in imminent danger, a parked car is extremely useful to keep distance between you and the attacker, particularly if you can't run fast. Try to keep the car between you and make lots of noise while doing it so this gives you a lot more time and space.
- When walking past a stranger, keep yourself at a distance, out of range, especially if something looks suspicious or doesn't feel right.
- If you're waiting for a taxi or a friend or any place

where you're standing still, position yourself where you have the fewest blind spots, and where it's difficult for people to walk up behind you.

Public transport

- Chose a seat near the doors or the driver.
- If there is no seat and you have to stand then position yourself by an exit or somewhere you can clearly see an exit and your fellow passengers.
- Chose a seat near a person or group of people who appear trustworthy.
- If you feel someone is following you, tell the bus driver: slip them a note or type out a message on your phone.

Taxis and cabs

Taxis and minicabs are great and a safe way to get around if you choose a trusted company to book with and take the following precautions. Remember: **safety over convenience!**

Taking a quick snap of the number plate or screenshotting the details of your upcoming ride on your phone and sending them to someone you know is an important precaution, even if it's a known company.

- A personal safety app can be useful – there are loads of options. Some can notify loved ones of where you are, track your phone or even enable to you enter a code to notify the police discreetly if you feel you may be in danger.
- Keeping your head up and taking conscious notes of the route you are taking is a good idea – if you are

looking at your phone and distracted, the driver could take you to an unfamiliar place before you realise it.

- If the driver does start to take a route you don't recognise, don't be afraid to ask questions and do so confidently. Assessing the situation early could save your life. If they are non-responsive when you ask them and you feel like they are deliberately ignoring you, tell them to pull over immediately!

- If they are still non-responsive, going live on Instagram or doing a FaceTime call can cause them to stop the car and want to let you out.

Evenings out

Whenever I go out for the evening, I always prepare my journeys. I have travelled a lot for work and picked up lots of little habits that have saved me problems later when I have either been lost or something has come up that has changed the route of my journey. Below are a few basics:

- Charge your phone, and if you have a back-up charger, bring it!

- Familiarise yourself with the destination and the surrounding area. Where are the train stations, cab offices and useful bus routes?

- Tell someone where you're going.

- Pack a pair of flat pumps in your bag or wear them while travelling, and hold your formal shoes in hand – this is an option if your formal shoes are problematic to walk or travel in. If there is an emergency of any sort, you can move more easily to the exits. I have great balance, but I spend most of my time in trainers, so when I do wear heels I feel like I am on stilts, and my feet hurt so much by the end of the night that it's painful to walk, so I pack my kung-fu slippers (to my friends' amusement) because they are flat (I can even roll them up), and I will walk home in them. If my path is crossed by a perpetrator, then my heels are in hand as a back-up equaliser in a dangerous situation.

Hotels and overnight stays

- Do your research: check reviews and go to websites like Hostel Geeks before booking – they can provide links to female-only hostels, five-star hostels and safety tips.
- Choose locations close to city centres.
- Book hostels through reputable websites. They do the legwork for you and are all very safe.
- Don't be gender specific when booking your stay.
- Request a room that isn't on the ground floor.
- Ask the front desk to write down your room number so it is not announced for others to hear.
- Always forward copies of your passport and travel tickets to yourself as well as keeping a printed copy to hand.
- Check if your door locks and then always lock your door.
- Don't open the door to strangers, especially if you are not expecting anyone to knock. Treat your hotel door like you would your home front door.
- Look out for markings outside your room or door and see if there are any others around the building. Human traffickers often mark rooms or buildings. If

you see anything suspicious like this, leave
immediately.
- Inspect your room as soon as you arrive: there have
been growing reports in recent years of hidden
cameras being discovered concealed in ordinary
objects such as smoke alarms, clocks, wall sockets or
phone chargers.[5] If you think you see a camera, turn
on your phone flashlight and hold it directly at the
area. Cameras will reflect a red light. You can also
turn off the lights and scan the room with camera
flash to see if anything reflects back. You can also
download an app that can scan for frequencies.
- Check for two-sided mirrors. For these to be effective
they need the lighting on the side you would be
standing on to be ten times brighter than the other
side. If the light is dimmed you can usually see
through them so turn on lamps and turn off the main
lights and have a look. Hold the flashlight on your
phone up to the mirror and if it is two-sided you
should be able to see something beyond the glass.

SAFE

SAFE is a handy acronym for remembering some of the points we've
covered in this chapter:

SHOW UP FOR YOURSELF

Remember to show up for yourself just as you would a friend or
loved one. Put your safety first, before peer pressure, and before
the convenience of others. Know that you can choose to say no – to
another drink, or to any situation that makes you uncomfortable;

you can decide when you want to leave, and you can make your own decisions on how you travel.

AWARENESS

When you are out and about make sure you are aware of your surroundings. Be aware: use your eyes and ears, don't rush, minimise distractions and listen to your intuition. Remember that being aware is not the same as being on high alert; it is about being present.

FLAGS

Learn what they are and what to do if you meet someone demonstrating them:

- You keep seeing the same person in different locations.
- You get an uncomfortable feeling around them.
- Unwanted touching and attention.
- They don't respect your boundaries – 'No' is a full sentence.
- Trust your own intuition.

EXIT

If you feel uncomfortable, know that it is okay to remove yourself from the situation, even if that means changing your mind. If you feel you are in danger, take the nearest and safest exit and run to the closest public space or trustworthy person and tell them immediately what has happened. Contact the police. *Do not wait around* once you have a chance.

4.

FIGHT/FLIGHT/FREEZE

UNDERSTANDING OUR BODY'S RESPONSE
TO DANGER AND HOW TO REGULATE IT

Among the majority of women I have taught over the years, freezing has been one of the most common fears they have shared with me. It was also my fear, and a state I found myself in on many occasions. During my early days of training, I found myself in constant survival mode, and when faced with things like sparring my initial response was always to freeze.

I later found out that this was because I had an enhanced and overactive response to perceived danger – I would even perceive something mildly uncomfortable as a threat, such as when doing things that made me nervous. I literally felt terror when I performed martial arts in front of crowds early in my training. It was more than just feeling a bit nervous, and even though I knew I was not in real danger, I couldn't seem to switch it off.

My first time sparring for an advanced grading, I was put with my training partner, who was lovely but also a six-foot-tall man. And it happened again! I froze, had tunnel vision and just stood there. I heard a voice from my teacher to move, so I stepped forward – and that's all I did, so I was kicked, and I subsequently landed on my head.

There were no mats and I landed on the hard, very slippery floor.

The sparring was paused and I was given a moment to see if I was okay and to compose myself. I went and sat in the toilet, overcome with emotion. My hands were shaking, I felt dizzy, my heart was racing and the tears would not stop. I was feeling angry, upset, stupid, useless, humiliated and regretful that I'd ever wanted to do this. I managed to complete the task (badly), but I was shaken up the entire night, and that was the first time I nearly quit.

As awful as that experience was, it led me on my journey to discovering *why* I froze like that. The lack of sparring training was a factor, but my partner had the same training as me, yet it was me who froze and felt their limbs turn to jelly. I later learned that this immobilised state was likely because my automatic nervous system (ANS) was out of whack and basically not functioning properly, and that this was all due to my past traumas.

So, you can see how important it is that we understand the impact trauma has on our automatic nervous system, because the *why* and *how* lead to understanding *what* can be done to regulate it. If you are not able to compose yourself under pressure, or when a real threat is presented, it will be difficult (as I found) to execute a response to an efficient level, even if you train all the time.

The physical training is vital, of course, but it is not enough on its own. The ancient martial arts knew this, which is why their practices always married the physical, the spiritual and the mental. This approach works well for people who have a disproportionate level of aggression as well as those who freeze when presented with danger. Neither is a good response.

It is just as bad to hurt someone
who is not a threat as not to defend yourself
against someone who is.
KUNG-FU PRINCIPLE

In this chapter I will share with you my research and understanding of our physical response to danger, what I did to get the best results and how I eventually learned ways to overcome freezing.

WHAT IS OUR AUTOMATIC NERVOUS SYSTEM (ANS)?

Our ANS basically takes care of our automatic functions (heartbeat, digestion and body temperature). It also manages our survival and stress response.

As our ANS scans the environment it can produce three possible states in the body:

- **SAFE** – you feel calm, relaxed and connected to those around you).
- **MOBILISED (FIGHT OR FLIGHT MODE)** – the ANS detects danger and causes your heart rate and breathing to increase and the release of the stress hormones adrenaline and cortisol. Blood then rushes to your muscles so you can respond to a threat: either fight or flight.
- **IMMOBILISED (FREEZING)** – when the ANS detects that the danger is so great that you can't fight or get away, it shuts you down. In this state our heart rate and body temperature decrease and pain-numbing endorphins are released.

Throughout my years of teaching, I have noticed that certain types of people will go into certain states more fluidly: people who are 'approach motivated', such as extroverts and risk takers, were more inclined to approach a threat with a 'fight' response; people who were more 'avoidance motivated' were more inclined to have a 'flight' response.

But the ANS is not only used to detect danger. We also use it to navigate through the world each day, and if it is functioning well, it should move seamlessly from one state to another. If there is no danger it will combine the states; for example, when we are spending time with family it combines immobilised and safe states, and when taking part in an activity it combines mobilised and safe states. This helps us manage life and become resilient to stress and negative events.

If you have been exposed to trauma, however, or even chronic stress, it can keep the ANS from functioning in a healthy way and can often lead to us being stuck in a state of survival. This is where anxiety can creep in when we are doing everyday things, like having a meeting or socialising. We can experience threatening or frightening feelings, as in the situation with my grading, when ideally my ANS should have regulated my response in the 'safe and mobilised' state, but instead I went into pure survival mode.

Through my research I've learned that there is a whole spectrum of experiences that can have an adverse impact on the ANS:

- Shock or trauma – accidents, assault, natural disasters, war.
- Developmental/relational trauma: neglect, abuse, lack of safety as a child.
- Other – chronic stress, medical procedures, poverty, discrimination.

It's important to note that trauma is an experience and not an event. It's what happens inside of us as a result of something external happening to us.

....

Being in a constant state of survival has been linked to many chronic illnesses that are notoriously difficult to diagnose. I've listed some of them below.

Physical:

- Digestive disorders
- Chronic fatigue
- Chronic pain
- Migraines
- Autoimmune disease

Emotional/behavioural:

- Anxiety
- Depression
- Addiction
- PTSD
- Challenging relationships

All of these things contribute to a dysfunctional ANS, and when we have a dysfunctional ANS its scanning is broken and cannot tell the difference between our unsafe past and our now-safe present.

HOW DOES THE AUTOMATIC NERVOUS SYSTEM WORK?

You could consider the ANS as the traffic lights on the road that keep the traffic moving automatically. It has two branches:

- The sympathetic nervous system (SNS)
- The parasympathetic nervous system (PNS)

SNS = Green light = Mobilised state

The sympathetic nervous system operates your fight-or-flight response. When your SNS is activated, it switches on all the elements needed to minimise or escape perceived danger, drawing blood away from your non-essential functions, such as your reproductive and digestive systems, to allow for the flight from perceived stressors. A simple example is a racing heart when you are scared.

This could be seen as the green light in the traffic-light system, as it keeps you moving forward and puts you in the MOBILISED state. It does this automatically as a response to the visual stimulus (i.e. danger) that you are presented with.

The problem is, our modern lifestyles have us running on stress a lot of the time and this in turn keeps us in the fight-or-flight mode for longer than the SNS was originally designed for. It ought to be used only for short intervals, so continuous boosts of adrenaline can negatively affect blood vessels, raise blood pressure and increase the risk of cardiovascular disease. Further strain on your SNS can be caused by increased worry and fear, which makes it harder for your body to recover during rest. Imagine if the traffic lights were always green – it would lead to constant chaos on the roads.

PNS = Amber and red = Immobilised or safe states

The parasympathetic nervous system is responsible for your body's rest-and-digest response – the automatic response that tells the body it is safe – and works in opposition to your SNS to balance, calm and restore. It decreases your respiration and heart rate and increases digestion and immune responses. Unlike your SNS, your PNS is more easily controlled. So, for the sake of the traffic-light analogy, you could say that the PNS is like the amber and red traffic lights, reminding you to slow down and eventually stop (i.e. the IMMO-BILISED and SAFE states).

The control centres

The **vagus nerve** (VN) is the main component in the parasym-pathetic nervous system, which connects the autonomic nervous system with the sympathetic nervous system. It is the longest cranial nerve in the body, with branches that wander through your heart, digestive system, reproductive system and lungs. It's responsible for your internal organ functions as well as reflex actions (coughing, sneezing, swallowing and vomiting).

By branching throughout the body, the vagus nerve sends com-mands to the organs to either go GREEN (MOBILISED) or AMBER/RED (IMMOBILISED OR SAFE). It also carries sensory messages to and from the brain, releasing neurotransmitters into the amygdala.

The **amygdala** is the part of the brain responsible for the per-ception and regulation of emotions such as anger, fear and sadness, as well as aggression. It also helps to store memories of events and emotions so that an individual may be able to recognise similar occurences in the future.

Our amygdala is the alarm portion of our brain, and it forms part of the **limbic system**, a neural network that mediates many aspects of emotion and memory. It is constantly scanning for threats by recognising and gathering information around us. Using our senses, such as sight and hearing, the amygdala will respond with the feeling of fear if it perceives a threat.

If the amygdala sends a distress signal, the **hypothalamus** – a small but important part of the brain that controls hormone production – activates the sympathetic nervous system by sending signals through the **autonomic nerves** to the **adrenal glands**. These glands respond by pumping the hormone epinephrine (also known as adrenaline) into the bloodstream.

This all happens unconsciously, deep in our brains, and for the most part the process works well. The amygdala is great at its job, and at getting us to avoid danger – it's the thing that will make you move when someone swings for your head. But the problem is that it doesn't always know what real danger is. It can often interpret a perceived threat as a real threat – for example, we may feel anxiety or fear (triggered by the amygdala) when we are about to take an exam or speak in front of a room full of people. The amygdala can override our 'thinking brain', which is why, when we are presented with a difficult situation, we find we cannot think our way out of things. Our brain is wired to make us want to choose the easy option – to avoid pain, struggle and conflict at all. And sometimes this can make us stuck in a mental state of not wanting to deal with this at all, so we end up doing nothing: frozen in the mindset of avoiding the situation.

Emotional trauma and the amygdala

Studies have shown that PTSD affects the functions of the brain in multiple ways. The areas that are impacted by trauma the most are the **amygdala**, the **hippocampus** and the **prefrontal cortex**, which all play a part in regulating emotions and responding to danger.

Because the amygdala stores memory and is responsible for the perception of our emotions, it can become hyperactive or enlarged when affected by emotional trauma, often leading to a damaged or altered fight-or-flight response, which can leave the individual feeling extremely frightened or stressed even when they're no longer in danger. Often, stimuli can trigger overactivity in the amygdala if they are somehow connected to the traumatic event a person has suffered.

Depending on how trauma affects the brain, the person may be left with chronic stress, heightened fear and increased irritation. This might also make it harder for the sufferer to calm down or even sleep.

OVERCOMING FREEZING – THE 'IMMOBILISED' STATE

The freeze response is activated when you perceive the possibility of successfully fighting or running away as low. Survivors will likely have memories of times when they felt powerless, which make them believe that they cannot fight off danger or get away when they are threatened. It may be that their trauma taught them that it was easier and safer to be immobilised. This is common with those who have experienced childhood traumas or abusive relationships, where the individual's experience taught them that if they were quiet, agreeable or invisible, they could survive.

In nature, when a gazelle is brought down by a lion, freezing is likely to be the gazelle's only remaining possibility for survival. If it struggles, the lion will continue to maul it. However, if it freezes, the lion might wander off temporarily, giving the gazelle the chance of escape. I too felt like the gazelle for a long time; I felt defeated before danger even presented itself. It was a lie I was coerced into believing.

Now I turn to those of you who may feel similarly because of circumstances you've been placed in. You are not a gazelle. You can, in fact, retrain your brain and nervous system to respond with fight or flight, and you possess the same 'jaws and claws' that the lion does – you are a *lioness*.

It may sound silly, but the stories we tell ourselves from our past experiences are *so powerful* that they will impact on our belief systems.

If you believe that there is no other option but to freeze when danger threatens, your body will go into an immobilised state. It starts here, with what we tell ourselves. Remember: just because you once felt you couldn't defend yourself, doesn't mean you will never be able to.

This is why it's so important to first recognise *why* we are freezing, then learn what we can do about it while at the same time becoming aware of our own claws and jaws.

It's why knowledge of self-defence and self-empowerment must co-exist.

Exercises to decrease stress

Healing our nervous system can feel like a new beginning. And for those of you who have never experienced freezing or have never had past trauma, it's still useful information as the understanding alone of how the different nervous states guide our behaviour can help us become happier and healthier.

So below are a few things we can do to retrain our automatic nervous system:

Surround yourself with calm people:
- We automatically mirror the states of others, so those who are safe and attuned will reflect those states back to you.
- Give yourself the space to recover if you are around a friend who is always very stressed. Of course, we want to be good friends, but if your ANS is damaged then this can impact you more than others, so take the time to invest in self-care and wellness exercises.

Do activities that make you feel better:
For me, it was martial arts, ice skating, dancing, taking my son to Chessington World of Adventures or baking a cake with him. Whatever makes you *feel* better, give yourself the time to do those things. Even if it's just 10 minutes.

- Spend time in nature
- Yoga (see page 68)
- Dancing
- Cooking
- Meditation
- Martial arts
- Art
- Reading
- Chi kung (qigong) (see page 65)
- Riding a bike
- Gratitude activities (helping others)
- Critical therapies (If you have experienced trauma in your past, therapy will guide you through your healing. I am a real believer in the power of therapy. Just make sure you find the right therapist for you.)

All these things can contribute to your healing and help your nervous system become more regulated. And a regulated nervous system can *accurately* assess safety and danger and respond appropriately. We are truly resilient when we can fluidly move from one state to another.

Using martial arts to retrain your nervous system

'Lose your *mind* and come to your *senses.*' This is from one of my all-time favourite books, which I tend to read almost every year: *The Way of the Peaceful Warrior* by Dan Millman.

In the book, Dan is a young athlete who is highly motivated but very highly strung. His teacher, 'Socrates', keeps calling him a jackass because he says his mind is blinding him, and so he teaches him to connect with the now by encouraging him to come to his senses. It's a principle of martial arts that can help us to retain our nervous system and override the instinct to freeze.

Automatic reflexes

In my discipline we have an exercise called 'sticky hands', which is basically an exercise that cycles and repeats a sequence of moves in close and fast succession. This exercise trains your nervous system to have an automatic response. When executed efficiently, you do not even have time to think about a move, so you learn instead to rely on feeling and skin reflex. You end up losing your mind and coming to your senses. When I say 'lose your mind' I am referring to unhelpful thoughts; debilitating thoughts that can put you in a state of low self-confidence.

Bruce Lee said something similar: 'Don't think, feel.'

What this teaches you is that if you feel overwhelmed and fearful, you are distracted and not present. As we discussed in Chapter 3: Awareness and Planning, this may lead you to miss things, so pause, breathe and tune in to all your senses. Take note of what you notice through them.

A good martial art will have exercises to help you develop an automatic physical reaction – what's called a twitch reflex – as well as training you on tactics and how to think in a fight, include sparring. The good news is that once you train like this and you develop a twitch reflex, your confidence grows and you start having faith in your body's reactions. Having an automatic reflex is great when faced with danger because it overrides conscious thought. You are more likely to fall into the mobilised state automatically because you have repeated the moves over and over again, so your nervous system is now programmed to respond with them. It certainly overrides *my* conscious thought, and when caught off-guard my hands are triggered before my brain.

When I first experienced this, I was so elated. I began to notice that, because of my frequent training, my automatic response had become so ingrained that if I dreamt about punching, I would actually wake myself up because my arm would throw a punch!

Voice projection

If you have ever taken part in a martial arts class or even watched *The Karate Kid*, you will have noticed that they project their voices a lot with strikes, as well as counts – in karate this is known as *Kiai*, pronounced 'ki-eye'. This is because there is a connection between vocalising, shouting, projecting or screaming and opening our vagus nerve, which if blocked is linked to freezing.

There have been numerous studies on the benefits of screaming and voice projection. There are even cognitive therapies that use screaming as a tool. Singing and chanting can also be helpful. These studies have shown that people who scream or project their voice when lifting weights or striking experience an increase in strength of up to 7 per cent.[6] Pushing air out of your lungs through your mouth for a yell stabilises your core. It also helps focus your mind and reduce your fear trigger. This is known as a 'battle cry'.

Chi kung (qigong) – moving meditation

Chi (*qi*) means the vital energy and *kung* (*gong*) is the training of chi. Chi kung is an ancient healing practice that has been used in China for centuries to improve physical fitness and strength. Like yoga, chi kung focuses on meditation, breathing regulation and body posture. There are two types: dynamic and static. Dynamic chi kung involves the coordination of movements and meditation, and static chi kung focuses on mental concentration and body relaxation without physical movements. It is a common go-to for meditation for many martial artists.

Chi kung is also fantastic for those who struggle physically or have injuries, and it's something you can do at any age. A 2018 study by the School of Medicine in Taiwan[7] evaluated the acute physiological and psychological effects of one session of chi-kung exercise in older practitioners. A total of 45 participants with a mean age of 65.14 years were recruited, who noted that they felt less anxious and their body and autonomic nervous system more in balance after the session. When I went to China it was a common sight in the mornings to see members of the elderly communities in the local parks in large groups moving slowly through their chi-kung practices. It was beautiful.

In my own practice I was taught that chi kung can also increase your lung capacity, help regulate your heart rate, improve stress and anxiety and help with chronic illness and pain. It can also help you stay focused in stressful or intense situations. I can vouch for this myself, because chi kung helped me to manage some of the most intense situations I have ever experienced.

During the COVID-19 pandemic I lost four family members in fourteen months, three of them because of COVID-19 itself. This included the two main women in my life: my mum and my yaya. They died six weeks apart. Like many traditional Mediterranean families, we had three generations living together and sharing responsibilities. When our home was struck with the virus, everyone was sick apart from me and I had five people to care for, one of whom had dementia. It was the most extreme situation. On the day my mum was admitted to hospital, my aunt went into the same hospital within the same hour, and later that week my yaya followed. A mother and two daughters in the same hospital.

Chi kung literally kept me sane. It re-centred me throughout this awful period. Every time I felt immense fear kick in I asked myself those three questions I'd learned for interrupting fear: Who am I? Where am I? What time is it? (See page 14.) Even when I was called in to meet with the consultant I took a moment, slowed down my thoughts, breathed deeply and wrote down all the questions I had while in the waiting room. When they delivered the news that my mum's chances were slim, my heart broke on the spot, but I remained centred so that I could take in important information and deliver it back to my family. The consultant even asked if I worked in medicine since I remained so stoic. But being stoic does not mean an absence of painful emotions; I felt them all.

I still gave myself the space to cry when I needed to. Being centred in that situation meant that I did not go from one extreme to the other. I didn't allow myself to fall into false hope or let my fearful thoughts take over. My chi-kung practice enabled me to make decisions and feel things according to what was happening. At the time I couldn't predict anything – even the doctors said it was the most unpredictable virus they had ever seen. False hope would have had me falling hard if the worst were to happen, and fearing the worst would have meant fear running too high, so I was neither positive nor negative – just present. It was like sailing through an emotional storm. I managed to function even on the worst days. I even managed to organise and lead their funerals despite feeling the worst pain I have ever felt in my life. It had become so ingrained in me to breathe through the stress that I didn't even realise when I was doing it.

Basic chi-kung exercises:

1. Stand with your feet shoulder-width apart, knees soft, and feel yourself sink and connect with the ground beneath you.
2. Relax your hands and close your eyes.
3. Practise reverse breathing. Close your mouth, place the tip of your tongue to the roof of your mouth, breathe in deeply through your nose and as you do so allow your stomach to expand as you draw the air in. This allows your lungs to drop and frees up more space to collect more oxygen. Bring the focus of your breath to your dan tien, or energy centre, which is

found two inches below your navel, and allow your stomach to fill up. Do this as you breathe in and count to five. Breathe out through your mouth until all the air has been expelled from your lungs and bring your stomach in as you do this. Focus solely on the breathing and the count. If your mind starts to wander, bring your focus back to the breathing and the count.

4. Once you have familiarised yourself with the breathing technique, you can do a series of movements with your hands along with the breath; when you do this your focus should be solely on breathing and moving. This will help stop your mind from wandering and keep you in the present. The most basic movement is to draw your hands up from a relaxed position, keeping your middle fingers pointing towards each other and your palms up as if you are lifting something. Draw your hands up slowly and stop when you reach your solar plexus, then turn them over and slowly push them down. Lift up with the in-breath and push down with the out-breath. Do not let your hands touch.

Yoga

In the West, we are more familiar with yoga. Like chi kung it has many health benefits: it teaches you resilience, self-regulation and introspection, all of which give you the ability to understand what's going on inside your body. Yoga also regulates your nervous system by increasing vagal tone, which is your body's ability to successfully respond to stress. It is said that when your vagus nerve is toned and functioning properly your digestion improves, your heart functions optimally and your moods stabilise. You also find it easier to move from active or stressful states towards more relaxed ones. This enables you to manage life challenges with a balanced energy and engagement. You are considered to have a high vagal tone when you are able to consistently maintain this flexible state.

By continuously stimulating your rest-and-digest system, you start to rewire your brain to build new pathways of communication and find new ways to respond to certain stimulation. You can alter long-standing reactive behavioural patterns and therefore break habits of thought that don't serve you and destabilise your health. Take the time to find little intervals throughout your day to allow yourself to rest. Your body and mind will thank you, and you might end up being more productive and less stressed, and find it easier to get into the flexible state of mind that allows you to sway between SNS and PNS.

To help you achieve this, here are some tips from Elumi Yoga, based in South London, led by Eliza Ioannou, who is a member of the Fight Like a Girl self-defence team:

....

It's important to note that yoga is not only about postures (Asana). There are, in fact, eight limbs of the yogic path, and three of these – breath control (Pranayama), chanting (Mantra) and meditation (Dhyana) – can be particularly helpful in learning to access and control your parasympathetic nervous system:

1. Breath control (Pranayama)
The Sanskrit word *prana* translates directly as 'life force' or energy, and through the regulation of your breath, or pranayama, you can start to control or shift this life force or energy. This is one of the most accessible and effective tools to calm your nervous system, because you can do this anywhere.

For example, if you're on the train or in your car, on your way to work and stressed about a presentation or deadline, simply take three deep inhales and exhales. No one will notice what you're doing, and you might find that you feel slightly calmer afterwards. When you're calmer you're more focused, and when you're more focused you think more clearly and are able to react better to challenges, as you don't allow your emotions to get the better of you.

Sometimes repeating this action throughout the day is the easiest way to bring you back to the present moment. We can so easily be distracted, so it's nice have that little reminder.

2. Chanting (Mantra)

Scientific studies have shown that chanting can decrease stress, improve mood and help you to feel more relaxed and focused.[8] Even if you have never done chanting in a yoga class, consider for a moment how singing makes you feel. Perhaps there's a reason why singing is related to happiness …

Take a moment to try this exercise and notice how you feel afterwards. Lie down anywhere that's comfortable. Close your eyes or soften your gaze and take three deep inhales and exhales. Don't strain your breath. Take another three breaths just like this, but this time find a gentle hum on your exhales and focus on the centre of your chest. After your final exhale, stay there for another minute or so and notice how you feel.

This is a form of chanting, sending vibrations through your body and helping to activate your rest-and-digest response.

3. Meditation (Dhyana)

Meditation does not have to mean sitting with your legs crossed, hands in a mudra and your eyes closed. Meditation for you could be taking a walk in the park and being aware of your feet making contact with the ground; it could be you working in your garden; it could be you lying on your bedroom floor and listening to some soothing music.

Meditation is anything that allows you to focus your mind on one single thing. It's not stopping your thoughts or emptying your mind of all thoughts – that's impossible – but rather fixing your mind on a single point, noticing when your mind strays away from this point and bringing it back.

....

These practices have a cumulative effect and therefore the benefits can stay with you long after your yoga practice ends, or even permanently.

5.

RELATIONSHIP RED FLAGS

Even if you have picked up this book with the sole intention of learning the physical aspect of self-protection, this topic is a vital part of that journey, because statistically we are more likely to be exposed to violence by someone we already know.

The Femicide Census 2020 reported that:
- in 2020, 110 women were killed by men in the UK alone.
- of those women, 52 per cent were killed by their current or former partner.
- only 8 per cent of these femicides were committed by a stranger or where there was no known relationship between the victim and the perpetrator.
- 53 per cent of perpetrators had previous histories of violence against the victim or other women.[9]

With these statistics in mind, this chapter will include how to recognise the red flags in a romantic relationship, or in the behaviour of someone you may have declined a romantic relationship with, a friend, a colleague, a boss, or someone who is in your social circle.

A threat from someone you know can throw you, because we are more likely to feel safe with a face we recognise, someone we love or consider a friend, or even someone who was being nice to us at the pub. Familiarity can make us feel more inclined to trust – we might talk ourselves out of seeing the red flags, rationalise them, make excuses and tell ourselves we are just being paranoid – so it is important to know what to look out for, as it means we will be less likely to ignore those red flags and more likely to stick to our guns even when someone is being persistent. It can leave us prepared and ready to protect ourselves, emotionally, energetically and physically.

This is a form of awareness, because domestic violence doesn't happen overnight. It starts with a set of subtle behaviours that over time break down a person's self-worth. Manipulation and coercive control are signs of mental abuse and can often also lead to physical harm. Manipulators are very good at smoke and mirrors, so in this chapter we will look at ways to reveal the charlatans behind the curtain, as well as find your ruby slippers to get the hell out of there. Remember, our intuition often flares up to alert us of things our conscious mind has not picked up on, so do not ignore it. Check in with it and take it seriously.

This is a subject I really wish I'd had knowledge of in my adolescence. It has been a big learning curve for me. After several bad experiences, I wanted to discover how I could have been duped so badly when I was younger, and I realised there were so many signs that I disregarded because I didn't know what a controlling person looked like. I would just say, 'Oh, he is not controlling, just protective.'

Luckily there are some amazing organisations out there who have simple tips on how to spot these things. I have been so fortunate to have worked with such organisations and it has become a key part of the programmes I teach, as well as central to my own understanding, knowledge, and healing.

Bede House is a domestic violence service in Southwark that I have worked with and supported for several years now. They are dear to my heart, and their staff are a small group of incredible women. They attend my workshops and have shared their valuable knowledge on how to spot red flags – and they have given me permission to share these with you in this book:

RED FLAGS
(Provided by Bede House women's domestic violence service)

Cases where a perpetrator kills a current or ex-partner almost *always* start with coercive control, which is a form of mental abuse. The following red flags are very real indicators of a person's lack of self-control and their capacity for violent behaviour, and ways in which they can coerce another into being controlled.

Love-bombing: This is when a relationship jumps from the initial wooing stage to a fully-fledged relationship in an exceptionally short amount of time. Perpetrators will make themselves extremely comfortable in the lives of their victims and provide little space for the victim to digest what is happening or make an informed decision on their wants and needs.

Oversharing: Perpetrators often share intimate and private information about themselves very early on in the relationship to create deeper feelings of trust and intimacy. While some of this information may be true, it is often used to excuse abuse or in some cases pre-warn victims of abusive behaviour to place the onus back onto the victims.

Isolation: A common and extremely effective tactic used by perpetrators is to place themselves at the centre of the victim's life, cutting off support systems and independence – usually through speaking negatively about friends, family and colleagues, and advising that they no longer spend time with them. Often the perpetrator will pretend to have their best interests at heart.

How to notice these things, and what to pay attention to

The acronym **OAT** is a great reflection tool and a way to get you centred in the present so you can slow down and read the situation.

OVERWHELMING – Are you feeling overwhelmed by the communication of this person? Are you in contact more than you would like to be? Are you truly comfortable?

AUTHENTICITY – Do you feel yourself being pulled into a story or encouraged to share information about yourself too quickly? Are you being swept away by the story and the intensity rather than by who the person is and what they do for you?

TIME – Have you given yourself time to reflect on the conversations you are having? Have you allowed yourself the time to process any feelings you have? Have you given yourself time to figure out if you actually like them? Are you dating because of a pressure such as age, a big event, your body clock? Are these factors in your decision-making at all?

If you do feel overwhelmed, or that there is a lack of authenticity, or that things are moving very fast and you haven't reflected on it all yet, this is a good time to do that.

Other common red-flag behaviours to look out for

- Silent treatment – when it becomes a pattern it can be abusive.
- Gaslighting – trying to make you question reality.
- Belittling – trying to make you feel unimportant.
- Negging – often used by pick-up artists: making deliberate backhanded comments to their partner or flirtatious comments to another in order to bring the confidence of their partner down.
- Hoovering – an attempt to draw you back if they feel you pulling away. This is not changed behaviour; they will use love-bombing, lies, manipulation and threats of self-harm. They may create fake emergencies, spread lies, find ways to prompt you to contact them and make accusations to change the dynamic and try to get you to defend yourself.
- Inability to take on accountability or apologise.
- Lack of emotional control.
- Lack of self-control.
- Entitlement.
- Difficulty with rejection.
- Controlling – what you wear, where you go, what you spend, who you talk to.
- Manipulation.
- Objectifying women.
- Strong ideas about gender roles.
- Blaming you for their problems.
- Sexual narcissist – expects sex in return for gifts; gets angry at sexual rejection or not having their sexual needs met.
- Dog-whistling – when the abuser knows your triggers and mentions them in front of a group at a social event and presents it as a joke in the hope that you will react. They then have witnesses that you are 'crazy'.

Stalking

Stalking is often a precursor to physical abuse, assault, rape and, at times, murder. There have rarely been cases of those who have gone on to commit these crimes who did not stalk first.

Stalking is therefore a serious crime that often leads to even more serious crimes, so should you be experiencing it, please do not hesitate to report it to your local police force or contact the National Stalking Helpline for advice and support (see Resources, page 227). It should not be taken lightly. It is also punishable by law and, depending on the severity of the case, could lead to up to 14 years in custody.

It's a common misconception that stalkers are strangers to their victims; in fact, 45 per cent of people who contact the National Stalking Helpline have done so because an ex-partner or someone they know has been stalking them.[10] Being stalked can cause severe psychological distress, PTSD, anxiety and depression. It's important that it's reported, and that those patterns of behaviour are logged, whether from your own experience or that of other ex-partners they may have stalked.

Data from a report by the UK-based Network for Surviving Stalking suggested that victims' ages ranged from 10 to 73, included both men and women, and were spread across the entire socio-economic spectrum. The research concluded that anyone can be a victim of stalking,[11] although statistics show that the majority of victims are female (80.4 per cent), while the majority of perpetrators are male (70.5 per cent).[12]

What stalking looks like:
- Waiting at your home or place of work unannounced or uninvited.
- Persistent and unwanted contact that is causing you distress.
- Unwanted gifts, unsolicited letters and/or cards.
  Combined with other behaviours, and particularly

when unsolicited, this can lead to more intense forms of harassment. Keep anything you receive from stalkers as evidence – it could be used when making a case with the police and trying to make sense of patterns.

- Using social media to track you. Social media is becoming a more frequent tool that stalkers use to harass their victims and find out information on their whereabouts. Update your security settings, limit what you share online about yourself and report any contact you receive through social media and email.
- Finding an excuse to contact you. This could be after hearing that you are vulnerable – maybe you have lost a family member or broken up with a new partner. They try to disguise this contact as concern. If this happens after you have set a boundary not to contact you, this falls in line with harassment and stalking.
- Damaging your home, car or property.
- Spreading rumours about you.
- Making unwanted phone calls to you, whether sustaining a conversation or not.
- Calling your employer or school/university.
- Showing up or waiting at places they know you frequent. They may try to show this by posting pictures on their own social media to make it clear to you and your friends that they were in the same location as you. This can make you feel uneasy and should under no circumstances be viewed as normal behaviour.
- Using other people as resources to investigate your life, such as looking at your Facebook page through someone else's page or befriending your friends to get more information about you.

WHAT IS CONSENT?

Consenting to someone touching you in a sexual manner means agreeing to it by choice and having both the freedom and capacity to make that choice.

It is *not* consent if you or someone else was:

- Asleep, unconscious, drunk, drugged or on drugs.
- Pressured, manipulated, tricked or scared into saying yes.
- Not given the freedom and capacity to make that choice (e.g. because they were underage or a vulnerable person).
- 'No' is a full sentence. You do not need to make your case for refusing sexual or romantic advances.

HOW TO HELP A FRIEND

There are several things you can do if you are worried for yourself or for a friend.

— Clare's Law is a scheme that gives any member of the public the right to ask the police if their partner may pose a risk to them. It is named after the landmark case that led to it being instated. This scheme also allows a member of the public to make an enquiry into the partner of a close friend or family member.
— If you are in need of help or know someone in need of help, contact Women's Aid, Refuge or a local domestic violence service for advice and support.
— If someone you know is in need of help, listen, don't judge. Create a safe space where they are free to share without judgement.

I know from my own experience that I stopped talking about what was happening in my life because when I did the response was anger, and I was told to just stay away from him or leave him. It felt like people were angry at me, even though I know they were just worried for me, so I stopped telling people, and the quieter I became, the more isolated and the more embarrassed I was to tell them when things had escalated. I didn't want to feel stupid. The more silent I was, the louder the abuse became.

Be open to your friend changing their opinion of someone so they don't feel stupid. Avoid saying things such as: 'But I thought you said he was amazing.'

It's important to know that the signs are not always there at the beginning of the relationship. Abusers put on a convincing act at first to gain love and trust, and to form a bond very quickly. This stage may appear like a whirlwind romance from the outside; others may find themselves also thinking that this person is amazing and feeling happy for their friend. You can also keep an eye out for those key signs laid out in the OAT acronym (see page 76).

Without realising, sometimes we can have a kneejerk reaction to news we are receiving, so make sure you take your time before you offer a response and try not to let your emotions drive you.

Another damaging response is to try to make your friend feel better. The conversation may be uncomfortable, and no one wants to see their friend feeling sad, but be thoughtful and careful with the advice you offer. Try not to play devil's advocate in this situation, because you could unintentionally end up gaslighting your own friend. Avoid language like:

— 'Maybe he is just a bit jealous.'
— 'Did you communicate that with them?'
— 'Maybe he's just really scared of losing you.'

If your friend is in an abusive relationship, this sort of language is likely being used already, so it can be harmful coming from someone they like and trust. *Listen first* and create a space for sharing. Take your time before responding and avoid trying to give a solution.

Signs your loved one may be with an abuser

Below I've detailed some patterns you may want to keep an eye out for if you suspect that a loved one may be in an abusive relationship. It is important to note that while some of these occurrences are very strong indicators of abuse, such as suspicious bruising, they should not just be taken at face value. It must be more a case of noticing patterns and consistent behaviour, whether in the abuser or the victim. It is important not to make rush decisions as this is an extremely sensitive topic. If concerned, let your loved one know that you are always around to talk, and create a safe space to do that.

These notes can also be used as a means of self-assessment. If you notice any of these patterns in your own behaviour and your own relationship, you may want to seek advice or reflect on your situation.

- They are overly emphatic about how great things are, but you also sense sadness. Look to see how they are when they think no one is watching, or if you notice them gaze down at their phone and look sad or anxious, or find they look like they are deep in concerned thought.
- They ask your advice, but also question their own sanity, saying things like, 'I'm probably being paranoid' or 'I'm probably overreacting'.
- They are always checking in with their partner. Pay attention when you ask them to join you at an event.

They may look over to their partner immediately as though they are unable to decide for themselves.

- When you try to talk about your suspicions of abuse they avoid eye contact and display nervous and withdrawn body language. They may show signs of feeling embarrassed or shameful.
- They are over-defensive of their partner and make excuses for their behaviour. They may shift the blame onto themselves.
- They are always making excuses for why they cannot meet you and never have time for themselves.
- They are overly agreeable with their partner.
- If they share with you about their partner's abusive behaviour, they may insist you do not say anything to anyone about what you've been told.
- They may tell you about all their partner's 'crazy exes', how horrible they were and what a hard time they had. Abusers often tell their partners about their crazy exes so that when their victim tries to call them out on their behaviour, they can liken them to their 'crazy' ex.
- Their partner seems to always hold their money and your friend never seems to have cash or cards on them.
- They may seem uneasy in a social environment, as though they are constantly trying hard to appear a certain way.
- They may turn to substance abuse, such as alcohol or drugs.
- They may explain things that need no explanation.
- They may lose interest in their hobbies or other activities.
- They may drop out of school/university or start slacking off at work. They spend more time alone and at home.
- They may be hesitant when explaining what's wrong,

as if trying to look for a reason or excuse.

- They may report to their partner before making any decision.
- When their partner makes a joke, your friend may show a pained expression but laugh and find an excuse to leave the room.
- They may develop low self-esteem and show signs of depression.
- They may have erratic mood swings, such as sudden sadness or anger.
- Your friend may behave out of character, but their partner appears vibrant and charming when arriving at a social gathering.
- They may shrink when their partner enters the room.
- They may suddenly start adhering to very traditional sex roles, which is all the more concerning if that's not what your friend wanted before the relationship.
- They may tend to their sulking or angry partner instead of enjoying a social gathering.
- They may get nervous if their partner drinks or uses other substances.
- The may go overboard to make their partner look good.
- They may stop taking care of their own mental, emotional, physical and spiritual needs.
- They may have visible bruising or marks, or consistently wear clothes that could hide bruises.
- They may withdraw from other platonic relationships, social events and family gatherings, and cut off communication.
- They may say they hate their partner one day and feel empowered to leave, then make their partner out to be a saint the next time you talk.

Signs of abuse in your colleague

- They never attend company parties and avoid socialising with most people (especially the opposite sex). They may seem defensive or fearful when explaining why.
- They often appear upset at work or you can tell they've been crying when they leave the restroom.
- They spend most of the workday whispering into the phone.
- Their partner shows up at work and your colleague reacts strangely.
- Their workday is often interrupted by 'family emergencies'.
- They become overly anxious about leaving work late, especially when it is a last-minute decision.
- They seem forgetful and distracted, as if they aren't mentally present.
- They take sick days frequently.

Spotting the abuser

- They may steal the show when the victim has the chance to shine, or on the victim's birthday, a favourite holiday or an anniversary. And they may find a reason to pick a fight on these occasions.
- They may be jealous or paranoid.
- They may belittle your friend, lie about them, attempt to make them doubt themselves or change your friend's story to their own version.
- They may talk as if they rescued your friend in some way, from themselves, or from their last job or

relationship. Due to low self-esteem, your friend may find themselves agreeing.

- They may mention your friend's substance abuse problem derisively but not act in a compassionate or caring way. They may use the addiction to blame your friend for anything.
- They may seem too good to be true.
- They may flirt with you but deny doing so.
- They may be overly concerned with image.
- They may confide in you about your friend's supposed problems, which you cannot imagine being true.

Above all, when looking out for your friends or for yourself, *always* trust your gut.

6.

ASSESSING A THREAT

Assessing a threat gives you the ability to know when to do what. I have had the same question pop up in my courses over the years and that's: 'What if I escalate things?' This is a valid and important question. However, what if it's already escalated? Knowledge is power, and that power can give you the right answers to the situation you find yourself in. If someone is a low-level threat and you did not read that and went on to punch them, what could have been managed by simply ignoring someone or using words has now escalated. Similarly, if the situation has escalated to the point where you are in physical and imminent danger and you do nothing because you are worried to escalate it further, this may leave you in greater danger. This chapter covers knowing when and how to take measured actions.

In previous chapters we have looked at awareness and relationship red flags. We have learned about certain behaviours that indicate abuse, as well as how to spot threats early through increasing our awareness. **This chapter is all about how to *assess* what level of threat a person poses, and the appropriate level of response from you.**

Not every person is a high-level threat, or a real threat at all, and having the ability to determine that can leave you feeling at ease as well as prepared. Some unwanted interactions can be managed simply by ignoring them, setting a verbal boundary or setting physical boundaries either with disengaging techniques or by repositioning ourselves.

Self-defence is not only about defending against physical advances; it's also about knowing how to use dialogue, set boundaries and communicate without conflict *when appropriate*.

Before I learned *when* to do what, I felt anxious, caught between hesitation and feeling like I needed to be constantly prepared. Even though I knew quite a lot of moves, not knowing when or if a person posed a threat left me uneasy. I didn't want to hit someone when the situation just needed dialogue, but I didn't want to be caught off-guard either. So knowing *how to* defend myself without knowing *when to* still posed a problem.

There is a kung-fu principle that says it's just as bad to hurt someone when you didn't need to as not to hurt someone when you do need to. And as with everything in kung fu and in this book, it holds a double meaning. It's not just about the physical aspect. A threat can also be an emotional one.

HOW TO ASSESS A THREAT

To assess a threat, we must first understand the different levels of threat, and what response is appropriate to each level. It's important to note that your response or course of action should be based on your *honestly held belief* of what kind of threat you are facing. For instance, a person may only be verbalising their threat, or their actions may indicate a high level of threat despite not acting on any of it yet. If you honestly believe that they pose a serious threat based on what has been said or done, then you can alter your response based on that. You do not have to wait for a person to start physically harming you before you respond.

Who is the perpetrator to you?

Thinking about this is so important. The behaviour of someone you know may not be as severe as someone you do not know, but it may still present a high level of threat. When looking through the levels of threat it's important to imagine the following possible scenarios:

1. Someone you know

This could be someone you already deem a threat, someone you are unsure of, someone you may feel uneasy around and are not sure you can trust, or someone who consistently finds ways to overstep your boundaries. If that person seems to keep appearing where you are, approach the situation with caution, particularly if you're getting a bad gut feeling. Even if it appears that their presence is just a coincidence, if you feel uneasy and you know this person may be a danger to you, and has demonstrated those behaviours in the past, then the level of threat is potentially high.

It's sometimes a lot harder to set boundaries with someone we know, trust or like, or someone we are already afraid of but we overlook their behaviours or just want to avoid them. I invite you to take a moment to reflect on this.

2. Someone you do not know

This is someone you have never met but who you encounter while you're out. This person may call you over but you ignore them and carry on walking. They may persist and start to walk up behind you. Maybe they keep appearing along your journey, or maybe they have stopped you in your tracks to force you into dialogue. They may have been following you on your journey, and you notice this, and notice them looking over at you a lot. They may not even say a word, but it's clear they are in some way watching your moves. All these are examples of someone who doesn't respect boundaries.

The five levels of threat

Threat levels can change very quickly and do not necessarily follow in order. The levels are laid out below in order of severity so it is easy to remember what to do and what to look for, and to know what response is appropriate and best for you. For example, a Level-2 response would not suffice for a Level-4 threat. And similarly, a Level-4 response to a Level-1 threat would not be proportionate. This method of assessment allows us to find the *appropriate* solution.

Each summary includes examples of behaviour at that threat level and the appropriate response. Knowing what action to take at each level will allow you to be more prepared if the situation escalates.

Level 1 – Low: Unwanted verbal engagement, such as catcalling or saying things from a distance. **Action:** Ignore or use dialogue.

Level 2 – Mid/low: Dialogue in close proximity, online harassment such as unsolicited messages and photos, and invading your space, including touching, following, watching. **Action:** Manage by disengaging, space-managing techniques and setting boundaries.

Level 3 – Mid/high: Imminent physical danger – it's become apparent they are about to become physical with you by pursuing you or advancing towards you in an aggressive manner, expressing their anger or what they intend to do (whether verbal, online, by phone or letter), or grabbing your clothes and/or body. **Action:** Use of force that is reasonable and proportionate to the situation.

Level 4 – High: It is clear they intend to physically assault you and you honestly believe this is to cause you serious harm (grab, hit, pull, etc.). **Action:** Use of force that is reasonable and proportionate to the situation.

Level 5 – Severe: You have an honest-held belief that this person intends to severely harm you (life or death). **Action:** Whatever action is necessary for your survival.

....

In the following chapters we will break these levels down further and look at what you can do in practical terms to take the appropriate course of action in response.

SETTING BOUNDARIES TO ASSESS THREAT

It's incredibly important to note that how a person responds to you setting a boundary says a lot about their character. People who approach you to talk to you because they like you are not always a threat – a lot of the time they are trying to get to know you. However, if you are not interested, are not comfortable and do not want that engagement then that should be respected. People need to read the room. Being persuasive is no longer considered charming; societal standards have changed and being relentless in your advances towards someone who has said *no* is considered harassment. So, it's okay to set boundaries – you do not owe anyone your time, number or smile just because they decided to talk to you.

If we are receiving unwanted attention and our attempt to ignore it has not been respected, it's important that we set further boundaries, not in the hopes that they will listen, but because a person's response to those boundaries will give you an insight into what they are likely to do, if you can trust them and if they are a threat or not.

When it comes to cis-male versus cis-male interactions, the more attention they have from onlookers the more pressure they feel to fight each other. In contrast, men who target women or marginalised genders often view the situation as predator versus prey. When in this situation, the predator does not want attention from others; they want their prey to be isolated, scared and distracted.

Setting a boundary, verbally or physically, changes that dynamic. They will now know that you are aware of what they are doing and that you are setting out what is unacceptable and making any onlookers aware of this unwanted interaction too. Do this with the objective of *assessing* their response as opposed to *stopping* their behaviour. The stopping may be a welcome side effect, but even if they do not stop you are still left better prepared about what options you have to defend yourself.

A person is far more likely to respect a boundary if they are not *asked*, but rather *told*, as this makes them fully aware of what you will or will not accept. This is because you are taking control of what you will or will not do (e.g. remove yourself from the situation, end the conversation, hang up the phone …), as opposed to trying to control what someone else does or doesn't do. When you ask a person to stop doing something they feel they have been awarded the power to decide, whereas a boundary is an outline of what you will and will not accept, and the consequences of overstepping that. It's a far more empowering way to set a boundary, and whether they respect your boundaries or not will help you accurately assess how much of a threat that person poses.

SIGNS OF LOW-LEVEL THREAT

It's important to be able to recognise the behaviours that constitute low-level threat, as they require a much less aggressive response than high-level threats but still require decisive action. As a reminder, below are some behaviours that fall into Levels 1 and 2:

— Unwanted attention with non-aggressive tone
— Shouting things at a distance

— Catcalling
— Saying something insulting but with a non-aggressive tone about your appearance
— Touching, following and invading your personal space
— Online harassment
— Ignoring and not respecting boundaries you have set

In the next chapter we will explore the appropriate responses to these behaviours.

SIGNS OF HIGH-LEVEL THREAT

Below are some of the key signposts that indicate when a perpetrator has crossed the line from low-level threat to high level and poses a serious risk. These behaviours fall into Threat Levels 3, 4 and 5, suggesting imminent physical danger.

Violent language: They have verbally indicated their intentions; their use of language is extremely violent; they are using hateful words that indicate they do not value or respect you as a person.

Hate speech (racism, sexism, homophobia, personal vendetta, religious bias): Someone who is expressing hatred towards others based on who they are, how they look or what they believe in a violent, aggressive manner should be taken very seriously, and you should take necessary caution.

Incoherence: The person may seem highly agitated; they may mumble and say things under their breath or show signs that they will not respond to reason. In some cases, this may mean that the person is mentally unwell. That is not to say they are definitely a threat, but it is important to distance yourself if you feel unsafe. If you suspect that the person may be in mental distress, it is always best to contact a professional to help them.

Physical signs that someone is likely to become violent

Physical aggression is usually accompanied by physiological symptoms. Below is a list of signs that a perpetrator is about to attack. Even if they are not showing these physical signs very clearly, if you believe that you are in imminent physical danger, you should prepare to protect yourself and get to safety accordingly. Do not leave it to chance.

- Clenching their fists
- Lowering or spreading of the body
- Redness in the face
- Rapid breathing
- Lowered brow
- Showing their teeth
- Scowling or sneering
- Muscle-twitching
- Sweating
- Swallowing
- Dilated pupils
- Concealing their hands
- Looking over their shoulder

Threat Levels 3, 4 and 5 all require the use of force, self-defence techniques and survival tactics. They can escalate from mid-range to severe very quickly. When these signs are present, you will need to take any action necessary to protect yourself, and the following chapters will go into detail on how to do this.

7.

RESPONDING TO THREAT

LEVELS 1 AND 2: LOW-/MID-LEVEL THREAT

Threat Levels 1 and 2 are classed as low or mid/low level. Maybe the perpetrator is not showing indicators that they wish to physically harm you, but that does not make it okay or socially acceptable. You should not feel obliged to respond, but if you do feel the need to take action, these behaviours are deemed to require a non-physical response that will not escalate the situation, namely ignoring, distancing and setting boundaries. A low threat is not zero, so still be cautious. It may be considered low in terms of risk of physical harm, but if it's unwanted attention, it is still harassment and should be taken seriously.

Online harassment – course of action

If someone is harassing you through technology then you should set a strong boundary telling them to cease all contact. Harassment through technology, either through social media, email or text, is a criminal offence and can be just as damaging to our sense of safety and our general wellbeing as in-person harassment. Tell the perpetrator you will no longer be answering any correspondence, and if they continue then you will be contacting the police. If you have been explicit in setting your boundary for no contact and they break this and continue to try to contact you, this is harassment. Make sure to block them on all outlets:

- **Social media:** Remove and block them from all social media platforms. This ensures they have limited or no access to your information and your whereabouts.
- **Phone:** Stop answering their calls or texts and block their number.
- **Email:** Screenshot or print out the emails as evidence and block their email address, and make an official complaint or report it to the police if necessary.
- **Revenge porn:** This is the act of sharing intimate images or videos of someone either online or offline, without their consent, with the intention of causing distress. It's also known as non-consensual pornography. If you find out that someone has posted something about you online to draw you in (this may be a picture, private content or an attempt to smear you), fight the urge to contact them and report it instead. Take screenshots and get anyone you know who sees it to do the same before you report it to any social media sites or the police, as once its down you may lose the evidence of the crime.
- **Evidence:** Keep a record of everything and flag it all to the appropriate channels. Keep copies of any messages, log all attempts to contact you and note down the names of any people who have witnessed the harassment. Seek help from the police, a harassment lawyer or specialist organisations such as

Protection Against Stalking (see Resources, page 227) if the behaviour continues. These behaviours are indicators of a potentially dangerous person.

In-person harassment – course of action

Adopt confident body language

We already know from Chapter 3: Awareness and Planning that small changes to our body language can make all the difference to our confidence. A perpetrator is often looking for someone who probably won't put up a fight, so when confidence becomes visual they will see this and might be deterred. Nonetheless, I feel it's very important to emphasise that this tactic is to empower *you*, not to try to control their actions. This is a much healthier mindset to adopt, because ultimately we can only control our own thoughts, feelings and actions. It just so happens that, as a possible side effect, it could also deter a perpetrator. Below are some reminders of how to adopt empowering body language and positioning:

- Keep your shoulders back.
- Keep your head up.
- Swing your arms a little when you walk.
- Maintain a composed and strong demeanour.
- Keep your hands along the centre of your body. You can hold them in a non-threatening way but ensure they are central to your upper body so if you need to protect yourself, they are already there.

Increase your awareness

Again, as discussed in Chapter 3: Awareness and Planning, you should try to maximise your awareness of the situation and your surroundings where possible. If you are wearing headphones, lower the volume so you can hear the perpetrator. Be aware of where they are and walk towards a safe space.

BEING FOLLOWED

If you feel or see someone following you, this is a higher level of threat. If there are people around, ask them to pretend they know you, or walk into a shop and speak to the security guard, shopkeeper or anyone you feel can help you. Do not be afraid to alert others or ask for help. It's better to do this than to just ignore it and hope for the best, particularly when you have someone following or coming up behind you.

Ignore the talking tactic

Often perpetrators use language to try to encourage you to feel calm and familiar with them. They may tell you a story with lots of detail and can be very charming and convincing. They might try to get you to help them or follow them somewhere, or they might try to guilt-trip and manipulate you. This can be done by saying things like, 'Oh, so you're too good for me, eh? I was just trying to be nice.'

This is manipulation and people often respond to it – I was one of them; I never thought I was better than anyone, so I was hooked into a dialogue to try to make the person feel better about my no. Now I see this tactic for what it is – a ploy to distract, engage, insult or boost their self-esteem – so I simply do not care if they think badly of me for walking by.

Know that you are not obliged to respond to or reward anyone for 'being nice', particularly if it's an unwanted advance. You do not owe anyone your time or energy, and this does not make you full of yourself; it means you are in tune with your own boundaries, and that is a form of self-love. If you do not want to engage with someone then do not. A person's words, gifts, advances and attention (wanted or otherwise) are not a currency that can be used against you.

If you feel something is off, stay present! Don't allow yourself to be distracted by their words. Breathe, keep your head up and stick to your guns. If you feel charged with an emotion, then wait for it to pass before making any decisions.

Set boundaries

When I have taught my women's self-defence programmes a common concern that comes up is the potential to make things worse by engaging. This is a valid concern, but often we have to communicate a boundary with the potential perpetrator in order to assert our own agency and also to assess their next move. It is less about trying to change their behaviour, and more about making ourselves better prepared and more empowered.

I never used to set boundaries when it came to what I deemed low-level threat because I was worried about offending people, and it always left me feeling uncomfortable. But setting a boundary shouldn't feel like a confrontation; often, it only does so when it's set against someone who doesn't respect the boundaries of others. So now I always set boundaries, and most of the time they are noted and not crossed again.

How to set verbal boundaries

Use your voice: Set the rules in a strong, clear voice – not shouting, just using a strong tone with clarity and composure. This allows you to communicate the boundary effectively and still maintain the element of surprise. Tone of voice is everything in communication: people generally take more notice of tone than they do words. Using a commanding tone has several benefits:

- It boosts confidence within yourself.
- It alerts others to the situation.

- It gives the impression that you are not afraid to stand up for yourself and therefore not what they perceive as an ideal victim.

Attack the behaviour, not the person: Avoid name-calling or personal attacks as that may escalate the situation. Maintain a strong and assertive tone, directly addressing the action. Remember to tell, not ask, and confirm what you will not accept. For example:

- 'You are sitting too close to me.'
- 'Stop approaching me at my desk.'
- 'Stop sending me gifts.'

How to set physical boundaries

If a person has invaded your personal space but you do not believe it is a high-level threat, using force or striking them would be a disproportionate response. The situation can instead be managed by using disengaging techniques (see below) combined with verbal boundaries (see above). Negative physical behaviours that may make you uncomfortable include:

— Touching or pulling your hand to get your attention.
— Standing in front of you to block your path and forcing conversation.
— Putting their arm around you.
— Going in for an unwanted hug.
— Unwanted touching of your hair, earrings or necklace.

Any of these actions may happen before dialogue, and even if it is clearly not a high-level threat – someone may grab your hand in a loud club because they think you can't hear them and are 'just trying to get your attention' – it is still crucial to set a physical boundary with any unwanted attention. The reality is that you don't know if they are a real threat or not, and if you do not set physical boundaries, you are less prepared to respond if they are a threat.

For instance, I once saw a guy outside a nightclub pull a woman towards him and as he was talking he was holding her tightly. It was clear she felt very uncomfortable, so she asked him to get off her, matching his aggressive energy. He escalated the situation, calling her a slut and speaking very closely in her face. She managed to pull her arm away and walk off, but she was visibly upset. Other girls, including myself, called him out and he responded by spewing insults at us and then walking off.

What if this had happened in an isolated place rather than outside a nightclub? He was demonstrating that he had the capacity for violence and took rejection very badly. If they had been alone, the woman could have been in a very dangerous situation. So even if you just feel someone grab you gently, if it's not what you want and you haven't given the sign that it is okay, it is better to react instantly and maintain control. Here are some techniques you can try:

Defence positioning: Let's say someone who you feel uncomfortable around has turned up at a social space you are in. You have experienced them violating your personal space before, so you want to be able to deflect any physical touching when that person is nearby. Keep your hands at the centre of your body, as this will allow you to move them to any other area of your upper body and more easily deflect any advances. It is where we set a guard if we do feel a more serious threat may be possible, but at this stage you can just keep them centred and relaxed, ready all the same. Maintain a good distance from the other person, and make sure they are in front of you, not to the side or trying to get to a blind side of you.

Disengaging/space-management techniques: Below are some helpful defensive techniques you can employ in specific scenarios when you need to physically disengage yourself from someone's unwanted touching and re-establish control of your personal space. Using these techniques means that your hands are prepared if the situation were to escalate.

Harassment disengaging techniques

If someone tries to grab your hand ...
This move is called 'the beggar's palm' because the palm lies face up, as if requesting money. It places you in a good position to control the situation should your opponent get aggressive. If the situation does escalate, you can use your other hand to strike them.

- Relax your wrist completely.
- Use your elbow to drive your hand forward, moving your fingers towards the direction of the other person's centre line (see page 120), towards their chest, throat and nose, for instance.
- Place your hand on top of their wrist to weaken their position.
- Once your hand is over their wrist, turn it face down, using the outside of your hand to apply pressure. Ensure that your arm is still facing forward and not sideways.

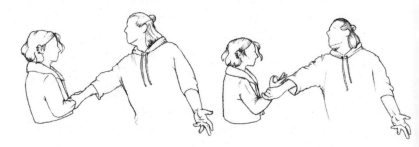

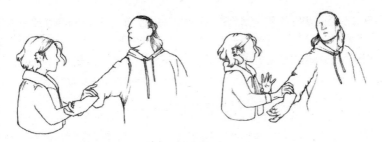

If someone tries to place their hand on your waist ...

This movement is illustrating the principle of having a 'rubber' elbow. In relaxing the elbow we do not need to raise it, or pull it back to reposition our arm; we can just hinge it to circle round the obstruction instead. This makes the disengagement move subtle, swift and less telegraphic.

- Corkscrew your wrist around the person's arm, going from the outside to the inside. Hinge the movement from your elbow – do not tense it; allow it to bend and be flexible as though made of rubber.
- Keep your other hand on your centre line (see page 119).

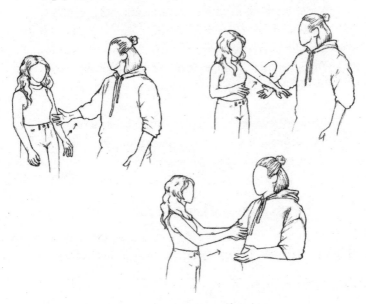

LEVELS 3, 4 AND 5: ESCALATING THREATS

Threat Levels 3 and above all pose a risk of imminent physical danger to varying degrees. If you have an honest-held belief that this person presents a physical threat to you, intends to physically harm you or has the capacity for physical violence, then use of force is appropriate but should be reasonable and proportionate to the situation.

Someone you don't know – course of action

This might be someone you are aware of, even if you don't know them – for example, someone you might have seen more than once on a night out, lurking nearby or showing up where you are, and it appears to be deliberate. This could be someone planning to target you. Or it might be a stranger trying to get a young girl or someone more vulnerable than they are to come with them or get in their car. They may use certain tactics, such as saying their car has run out of petrol, or they need your help in some way. In this scenario:

- Avoid interaction with them altogether if possible.
- Do not try to reason with them.
- Do not answer any of their questions or respond to guilt-tripping. Keep your distance and keep your hands at the centre of your body to protect yourself in case things escalate.
- Find somewhere safe and wait for someone to come and get you. If you feel the perpetrator is a real and imminent threat, call the police.

Someone you know – course of action

There are pros and cons to already knowing the person who is threatening you. You will have an insight into their motives and what they are capable of, but because they are also familiar, it can feel easier to interact or try to reason with them. You may feel the person is trying to guilt-trip you to get you to come somewhere with them, help them or interact with them, but it's important not to give in to those ploys.

- If they appear where you are, take this very seriously and approach with caution. Do not talk yourself out of being cautious or make excuses for why they might be there. From my experience, if someone has already demonstrated that they have ill intent, if they have a history of stalking and harassing you and they start appearing where you are, it's fair to assume it's deliberate.
- If you already know that a person poses a threat from past experience, follow the same advice as if you don't know the person.

....

You do not have to deal with harassment alone. Talk to people who can help. Most schools and workplaces have policies in place for help and support. If the harassment and stalking is not happening at school or at a workplace, you can contact the National Stalking Helpline (see Resources, page 227).

If the harassment or stalking is by someone you are or were romantically involved with, a family member or someone you were close to, you can contact your local domestic violence service. Further information on how to get in touch with various organisations can be found at the end of this book (see Resources, page 227).

....

Regardless of whether you know the perpetrator or not, so long as you have an honest-held belief that you are in physical danger, the level of response will be down to what you deem the level of threat to be (see page 90 for a reminder on the five levels of threat). For example, if someone grabs your clothes to pull you towards them, you may just use a self-defence technique combined with a strike to give yourself time to get away. But if that person is trying to drag you towards a car you might use a higher level of force to create more damage and give yourself more time to get away.

This level of threat will likely require the use of self-defence, including force, counterstrikes and causing enough damage to get away for the purpose of your own survival. You may need to fight back with anything and everything you have access to – this could involve using everyday objects or whatever you have to hand. Specific strategies and techniques for what to do and how to get to safety when posed with Threat Levels 3 and above will be covered in the following chapters.

8.

STRATEGIES AND TACTICS
(IMMINENT DANGER: PART 1)

The route to success in anything requires good strategy and tactics so that you can be more adaptable and know what to do and how to do it. Self-defence is no different. Strategy is the overall aim – in this case getting to safety – and the tactics are the steps that get you there. These include:

— Switching on your self-defence mindset
— Adopting a powerful pre-fight position
— Managing your distance and getting away if you can
— Using anything and everything around you to your advantage
— Using break-away techniques and strikes
— Learning the key self-defence principles so that you are efficient in all you do

Remember, the aim is always to create an opening, give yourself time and get to safety, never to go toe to toe with an aggressor, but if you are forced to defend yourself against Threat Levels 3, 4 and 5, you will likely need to use force and self-defence strikes to do so.

USE OF FORCE – IS IT OKAY TO STRIKE?

During my training I struggled with thoughts of getting into trouble with the law if I fought back, but a particular saying helped me disregard those thoughts and reminded me that they had no place in a moment when I really need to defend myself. The saying is: 'It's better to be judged by 12 than carried by 6.' In other words, do not let the thought of potentially having to stand up in court and give evidence as to why you needed to defend yourself hinder you from actually protecting yourself. Compare the situations: even if you did need to justify in front of a judge and jury *why* you needed to defend yourself, isn't that outcome still far preferable to the real possibility of death or severe injury?

It is useful here to first look at what the law actually says on this subject. English law currently states that the use of force must be reasonable and proportionate to the situation, and that a person may use such force for the purposes of:

- self-defence
- defence of another
- defence of property
- prevention of crime
- lawful arrest

Any use of force must, therefore, must be in a context of you trying to defend yourself or others. Revenge is not self-defence. To assess whether the forced used was indeed reasonable, the Crown Prosecution Service says prosecutors should ask two questions:

- *Was the use of force necessary in the circumstances, i.e. was there a need for any force at all?*
- *Was the force used reasonable in the circumstances?*

Both questions should be answered on the basis of the facts as the accused honestly believed them to be.[13]

When it comes to a pre-emptive strike, English law currently states that there is no rule in law to say that a person must wait to be struck first before they may defend themselves:

A person may use such force as is reasonable in the circumstances in the prevention of crime, or in effecting or assisting in the lawful arrest of offenders or suspected offenders or of persons unlawfully at large.[14]

So yes, it is okay to strike in order to defend yourself. I would urge you to check in with how you feel about that and to do some visualisation work if you find this concept difficult (see page 15). I struggled with this at first, but I am also a realist and know that a strike may be necessary in order to defend myself.

It's not a bad thing if you do not like the thought of hitting someone back; it doesn't make you meek or weak if you don't feel comfortable with the notion of causing another person harm. Most people feel this way. It is important to understand that striking to defend yourself and ensure your own safety doesn't make you a bad person. You have every right to protect your life and your wellbeing, and understanding this certainly does not mean you condone violence.

> *'Self-defence isn't violence;*
> *violence is fighting with the absence of justice.'*
> KUNG-FU PROVERB

I do not promote violence – I wouldn't even harm a wasp – but I also do not believe it's useful to just use a disengaging technique with no strike when the threat is high and the situation is dangerous. If a situation can be managed without the use of force then it should be, but if the threat is assessed as a high-level one, then you must have the capacity to do what is necessary to be safe. I see knowing how to fight someone off if needed in the same way that I view being prepared for bad weather. It's better to have access to an umbrella or a raincoat should the weather turn than to have no access to anything at all. You might not need it, but it's comforting to know that it's there.

Remarks like 'I don't believe in self-defence because I don't believe in violence' to me are unhelpful and misinformed, as the two are not synonymous. Preventing someone from causing you harm through self-defence is *anti*-violence. So please do not regard all use of force as a form of violence – it's more complex than that. *Violence is the use of force without the presence of justice.*

> *'It's better to be a warrior in a garden than a gardener in a war.'*
> CHINESE PROVERB

I have been there, I have seen violence rear its ugly head, and I did all the right things: I called for help; I ran into a shop; I tried to defuse the situation; I even tried pleading and apologising when I hadn't done anything to apologise for. On most occasions no one helped me, no one cared, and the perpetrator only became more violent and more confident. So having the ability to defend myself is now there as my back-up. I would never look for violence, but I do now have what I call 'a last arrow' if I need it, there for when all else fails, so that I still have the ability to defend myself.

THE SELF-DEFENCE MINDSET

To overcome any challenge you need to have the correct mindset. As explored in Chapter 2: Mental Discernment and Self-belief, in self-defence this is a vital component. Keep reviewing Chapter 2 and practise the tools there, particularly the ways you can interrupt fear and initiate the fight-back mentality.

Here is a simple strategy to trigger the optimum mindset in a defensive situation, using the acronym MIND to help you remember it. Note that this should be practised through visualisation first, as it's then more likely to be an intuitive response if you find yourself in a dangerous situation.

MIND

MANIFEST:

- Manifest your muse! Say out loud or in your head the words that connect you to your survivor instinct. For me it's 'lioness' or 'phoenix' as both are revered, capable and empowered; they embody all I feel I need to execute what I know. Alternatively, I think of protecting my son, so I manifest my motherly instinct. But this can be anything that gets you to connect to your fighting spirit and ignite the capacity to show up as your authentic self.

INTERNAL DIALOGUE:

- Interrupt any unhelpful thoughts that are telling you that you are incapable. Try saying the word 'Delete', counting down to interrupt fear or focusing on your anchor thought, and remind yourself that these thoughts are not true.
- Remind yourself, too, that you have the right to survive, you can find ways to get away and you can find a solution.

NEVER GIVE UP, AND NEVER GIVE IN:

- Agree with yourself that you will never give up on surviving, no matter how bleak things seem, how scared you are or how much the odds may be against you. This is particularly important when we are talking about a Level 5 threat. When your life is in danger, you cannot afford to become the gazelle. You don't necessarily need to physically fight back relentlessly, but you should not give up on using the strategies and tactics to help you out of the situation. You cannot just accept defeat – you must keep finding a way.
- When a situation feels hopeless, always know that there are people and organisations that can help you find a way out. Never give in to unhelpful, doubtful thoughts that keep you immobilised and in a state of giving up.

DECIDED:

- Be decisive in your actions.
- Hold the conviction of *knowing* you will and can get to safety.

> *'Our greatest glory is not in never falling,*
> *but in rising every time we fall.'*
> CONFUCIUS

PRE-FIGHT POSITIONING

When imminent danger threatens, you can physically prepare yourself for defensive action by positioning your body so that it's ready to both guard and strike. The first rule, of course, is to keep your distance and, if you can, find an exit and run. But if you cannot run and the perpetrator is already close or drawing closer, here are some steps you can take to ready yourself for attack:

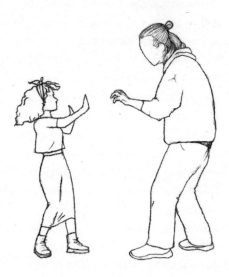

Protect your centre line

All the areas we want to protect the most are close to the centre of the body, so we must always hold our hands along the centre line of our torso to defend that area.

1. Hold your hands at the centre of your body, elbows bent, with one hand forward and the other in line with the elbow of your front hand. The line of your hands should be pointing towards opponent's nose. If they

are taller than you, your hands should move higher. This is your guard position.

2. By having one hand forward and one hand back you're giving yourself two lines of defence and more options to work with, because if one hand fails or is held, you can use the other. The perpetrator would need to get past the first and second lines of your defence to get to you. If you held up both hands parallel this would be easier for the perpetrator, and it would also leave you with a space in between them, giving the perpetrator direct access to your centre line.

3. Hold your hands in a strong but non-threatening way. You can make the stance less inflammatory by turning your hands more towards your opponent, as if to say stop or back off, as opposed to presenting an obvious fighting guard. We still want to maintain the element of surprise, though, and at this stage want to position our hands so that we are prepared for any strikes, grabs, pushes, pins or any form of physical violence, so I find this hand position is the best balance. It keeps you prepared, and if they do try to grab or touch you, you are better able to control your space.

4. Keep your hands fluid. Don't hold them out like a statue; instead, allow each hand to move as needed: if the person moves to your right, you can move your right hand or your strongest hand forward as well. Later you will learn how to use each hand independently, but it is important to keep them on your centre line and not to fix them in a rigid position.

5. Ensure the person cannot outflank you – keep your nose on their nose (see page 123).

Distribute your weight

Because we want to be able to move in any direction quickly, the distance between the legs is important. Everyone is different, so to find the ideal distance for you, I want you to stand up and put your feet in a neutral position like in the diagram below. Point your toes in just slightly so that your knees are protected. Keep your knees slightly bent and make sure your pelvis is tucked under. Now, with your legs in this position, I want you to pivot one foot so that you are turned 90 degrees to your right. If you can lift your turned leg up easily without leaning back then this is a good distance. If you find your front leg too heavy then the distance is too wide.

Shifting 45° and 90°

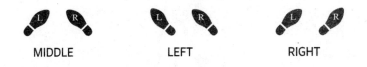

MIDDLE   LEFT   RIGHT

The turned position you create from pivoting your foot can also be stepped into if you need to move out of the way – of a larger person, for example – and a turn alone wouldn't suffice. This step is called the 'falling leaf', because as a leaf falls from a tree it falls from side to side on its way down. When we step this way we are simply moving from our neutral position to the turned position with a step to the side.

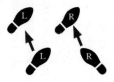

The neutral stance is also the position we need to adopt for our moving stance – the position you would be in once in motion. If I were to step from my neutral pre-motion stance into a step forward, it would resemble the step and turn, like this:

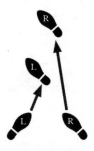

Your four distance lines of defence

Judging the distance between your field of attack and your opponent will help you know when to use which weapon. You want to ensure your strikes are not easily foreseen, so you shouldn't try to use an elbow when you are not in range, for instance, as it will be easily anticipated. Always look for what is available to you and what weapon is within the shortest distance between you and your opponent.

DISTANCE LINE 1: KICKING	DISTANCE LINE 2: PUNCHING, OPEN HAND, KNEES	DISTANCE LINE 3: ELBOWS, HANDS	DISTANCE LINE 4: BODY LINE, SHOULDERS, TURNS
Your legs are your longest weapon. The point where your kick ends is the line within which you can reach your opponent.	This is the line from your front hand in the guard position. Keep your hands pointing towards your opponent's nose with a bend in the elbows. Ensure your elbows adjust if your opponent's width is larger than yours. At this range, you can also use your knees.	Your rear hand will be in line with your front elbow in the guard position. From this line you can use your elbows, and you can also use your hands if your opponent is in this range.	This is very close range – maybe your opponent has advanced right up to you and you need to turn to deflect their strike, or your hands may be pinned to your body line (e.g. your opponent has grabbed you from behind over both arms, but you can still move your hips and your arms from the elbow down).

'A person who knows their distance can never be beaten.'
KUNG-FU PRINCIPLE

FIGHTING PRINCIPLES

Let's look at some of the fighting principles that underpin effective self-defence strikes:

Know your targets

As with any journey, it's good to know the destination or you might not like where you end up. The targets we are looking at when it comes to self-defence are very easy to remember: those closest to the centre of the body are the weakest. They are those that are not protected by muscle mass, height or width. When I first learned this it gave me confidence, especially when faced with much larger opponents.

When I'm introduced to people and they find out what I do I'm often told to follow the same old tactics by someone who is often feeling threatened by the fact that I may know how to fight. They always say, 'Just kick them in the nuts, then nut them in the face.' I always respond with, 'Oh, wow, yeah, I hadn't thought of that ...'

The problem is that the majority of people who say this are male, big or very aggressive. It's easy to kick someone in the nuts if you are already standing up against them, you have already used the tactic of intimidation and you have no fear of losing or getting hurt.

It's not so simple when it comes to fighting someone who is a lot taller and physically stronger than you, has a longer range and is very aggressive when you are not. Yes, a strike to the groin can be very effective, particularly for creating space to run away, but it's useless if your opponent sees it coming or you are not even in range.

Let's look at the weakest targets on the human body (see diagram below). The line right down the centre of the body is what we call our vertical mid-line or the meridian line – it's useful to imagine this line when we look at our opponent to find those targets.

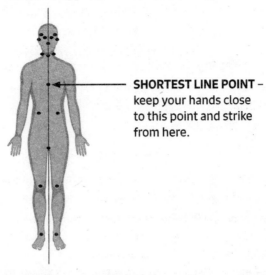

SHORTEST LINE POINT – keep your hands close to this point and strike from here.

- Eyes
- Nose
- Ears
- Throat
- Sternum
- Solar plexus
- Kidneys
- Ribs
- Groin
- Knees
- Ankles
- Toes and fingers. If you are struggling, cannot reach any of the main targets and the attacker is pinning you down, try to wrench or break their fingers.

Remember that the weakest targets on your opponent's body are also the weakest targets on your body. This is why we must always simultaneously protect our centre line (see page 119), strike from our centre line and attack the centre line.

Protect your centre line, strike along the centre line
and attack their centre line.
FIGHTING PRINCIPLE

Use the centre line

The centre line, where our and our opponent's weakest targets are, is the focal point of defensive action: it is the line we must protect, and the line where we must strike.

Strike from the centre line

Should you need to use force to defend yourself you want to make sure you do this with minimum effort and maximum outcome. Imagine a three-dimensional line between you and your opponent, from the centre of your body to the centre of theirs. This is the shortest, most direct line of attack, so this is the line you should strike. A straight strike from the centre of your body is one of the most difficult to detect and defend, and it requires the least amount of energy and effort from you. It will also reach your target more quickly, as your hands are already in place.

Attack the centre line

As all the weakest areas on the human body are close to the centre, this is where we must target any of our attacks as well as where we must keep our hands. And these must happen simultaneously. Your defences should be structured to allow the force of the attack to go in the intended direction while you move and use the force they deliver against them.

Use non-telegraphic moves

The best strike is one that is simple and that you cannot see coming, so not allowing your opponent to foresee your next move is vital. A non-telegraphic move is one that gives no forewarning, and there are various ways to do this:

— *Guard:* Because your guard position when you're protecting your centre line (see page 113) gives two lines of defence, it allows you to fire a strike from any hand without pulling back.
— *Hit from where your hands lie.* In other words, strike from where your hands or legs are; do not pull them back first, as this makes it easier for your opponent to see your next move and defend themselves. Your hands should be kept in front of your body, at your centre line, with your elbows low and bent so that they are ready to fire without having to pull back. This does not mean, however, that you should change where your hands are if they've caught you by surprise when they happen to be at your side.
— *Use the shortest and most direct route to strike.* This means using straight lines, not circular motions, when striking. We want to use moves that are the most difficult to detect, and circular or round moves (such as a round slap or a swing punch), though they can be good, are more telegraphic.
— *Strike from a low elbow position.* If your elbows are bent, you have range to fire from, and if they are low, it's more difficult to see the strike coming. Striking from this position also allows you to use the least amount of energy.
— *Keep your legs under your spine, and your head over your spine.* Where the head goes your body follows, so if you

leave your legs behind, you have little room to adapt and keep stable if the opponent moves or pulls you. By keeping your body weight behind the strike and your legs in line with your head (particularly your back leg), you can use your weight behind the strike.

— *Use small and subtle movements* when you step and turn.

Attack and defend at the same time

No one is going to stand there and freeze their punch waiting for your counter, so it's important to be able to defend and attack at the same time. This allows you to simultaneously protect your vitals and put your opponent out of action by striking their weakest targets. It's also more efficient: blocking alone and then countering afterwards is two moves, rather than one. And if you have not given a counterstrike after their first strike, they will likely throw another one.

Below are some examples of simultaneous attack and defence:

This is an example of defending a hook punch. One arm defends the punch, while the other strikes a weak target along the centre line, such as the solar plexus or the throat. This move also incorporates the wedge theory and the nose-to-nose method.

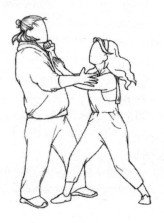

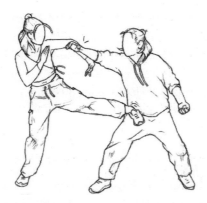

While deflecting a long-range punch, you can use a longer weapon – your leg – to strike.

The nose-to-nose method

This theory comes from a kung-fu legend about the female master Ng Mui, who watched a crane protect itself from a snake. To keep the snake from getting near and able to bite it, the crane kept its beak pointing right toward the snake's nose. Every time the snake moved, it moved too. The legend has many different iterations, but the lesson remains the same: if you think someone is about to harm you physically, you need to not only see them coming, but also make it difficult for them to outflank you or catch you off-guard.

Keeping your nose in line with their nose, as if there is an imaginary line between you and them, gives you this chance. Every time they move, you move too, keeping your body in line with theirs and your hands in the guard position, but maintaining the distance between you if possible. If your opponent is taller than you, lift your hands and head accordingly to line up with their nose – this is called covering your centre line.

The nose-to-nose method allows you to prevent an opponent from trying to be tricky and move around you, but if they advance forward with a linear attack, you can turn to defend against the strike.

This allows you to not disrupt the intended force and direction of their attack, while not being in the line of fire. When you turn you can use one arm to create a wedged shape to defend the strike and the other to counter (see below), but the turn is just as important. The nose-to-nose theory will also help you not to over-turn, but just enough to get out of the way.

Wedge theory

When you're defending a strike from a point of contact, the best way to deflect an oncoming and greater force than your own is to form a triangular or wedged shape with your defending limb, and the shape should be three-dimensional to enforce the structure. The fourth dimension is motion. If you move your arms horizontally outside your body lines to try to bat the strike away, you will be using the force of your arm only and your own timing judgement to do that. But by using this wedge shape to meet the oncoming force with a forward motion, you will be using the structure to naturally redirect the oncoming force. So instead of holding a strong, static shape with our limbs, we move them to meet the opponent's oncoming limb while maintaining the wedge shape.

How to create a good defensive shape with your arm:

1. Stand squarely in front of a mirror and bring the index finger of one hand to your nose.
2. Now move that hand in a straight line, pointing your fingers towards the nose of your reflection.
3. Keep both elbows bent low in front of your body, extending out in line with your shoulders, and roughly a fist's distance from your ribs.
4. Now turn your extended hand palm-down to face the floor, keeping your forearm flat. Keep your fingers pointing towards your reflection's nose, on the centre

line. This creates a three-dimensional shape, with your extended hand as the point of a triangle, and your elbows bent in line with your shoulders as the base. The height from the hand to the elbow creates a wedge shape. The forearm is what we will use to deflect oncoming attacks.

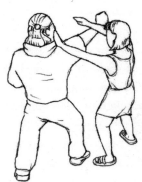

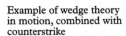
Example of wedge theory in motion, combined with counterstrike

Dynamic force

Dynamic force is the process by which energy from an action can lend something that weighs a certain amount a lot more power – in this case, our limbs. This simple clearing technique below shows how you can use dynamic force in two opposing directions to break free from an aggressor's hold.

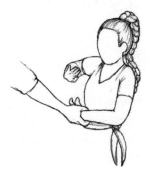
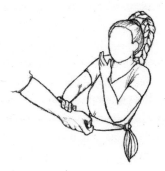

1. Relax both hands.
2. Slap down on the aggressor's wrist, firing your hand from your chest (centre line) and turn your body in the same motion (like a revolving door).
3. At the same time pull your other hand towards your chest, out from between their thumb and fingers – the weak point of an opponent's grab.

These motions together generate much more force and make the technique much more effective. The result can be very different, however, depending on how you apply that force. If you were to just place your hand on your opponent's wrist and push, with no dynamic force and no room for acceleration, it would produce a static force and lack efficiency. It simply wouldn't work as well, particularly against a very strong grab. If you were to do the same technical move with dynamic force, by giving the hand that's slapping down on the wrist some space, speed and acceleration, it becomes much more powerful.

The best way for you to generate dynamic force is to relax your limbs. If you hold tension you cannot generate enough momentum with your hand speed. Think of throwing a tennis ball. To throw it far and hard you need to relax your arm. The same applies to 'throwing' a punch; you are trying to transfer energy from your body into someone else's by throwing the power out, not holding it in. Firing from a low elbow position also helps generate momentum, because it keeps your body behind your arms.

TAKING ACTION

As stated earlier, your overall strategy is to get to safety, but you also need a strategy for each potential stage of a real threat. There may be elements of fighting within each stage, but this is all to create time and space to get away. It is important that you keep the overall strategy in your mind, so to remember it, use the below acronym below:

REACT

RAISE AWARENESS and **R**UN if you still have the space and time to get away.

EVERYTHING and anything around you is a weapon to create distance or help you get away.

ATTACK the weakest targets; if you're in close proximity, use self-defence, including strikes.

CALL for help, even if you have successfully defended yourself and got away. If no one has come to your aid already, call the police or shout for assistance.

TELL someone what happened as soon as you can. Having to defend yourself can be both frightening and traumatic, and this can lead to forgetting important details that are needed for arrest.

Below, we will break down each of these stages further, covering specific tactics you can employ.

RAISE AWARENESS and **R**UN
This is your first and best reaction when you have the time and space to move.

Make a noise
Making a noise and projecting your voice is a battle tactic and can:

- stimulate your vagus nerve, which in turn can leave you in a more mobilised state.[15]

- increase your strength by up to 7 per cent.[16]
- alert those around you.

Unfortunately, it's generally accepted that passers-by are less likely to go to someone's aid if they hear them screaming 'HELP!' or stop what they're doing and try to help if they think it's a 'domestic' or a physical altercation. This may be because they do not want to be harmed or because they feel that domestic assault is a private matter and do not want to get involved.

Nonetheless, it is crucial that you feel comfortable asking strangers for help. People are more likely to help if you speak to them. For example, let's say you run into a shop where you do make lots of noise, and say, 'Can anyone help me? Hide me, shield me.' You can hide behind counters, for instance. Be sure to tell security what is happening as soon as you run in, and shield yourself behind them.

If you are not in close enough proximity to anyone to explain the situation, you can try a strategic method to gain assistance. People are generally more likely to respond to calls of:

— 'FIRE!'
— 'I DON'T KNOW YOU!'
— 'STAY AWAY!'
— 'RAPE!'
— 'POLICE!'
— 'STOP!'
— 'AMBULANCE!'

Move or run

If you are able to run and find that this is the best option available to you in the moment, you should still make lots of noise in case they chase. Run to the nearest shop or anywhere busy, well lit and well populated. Do not run aimlessly. If running away is not a viable option for any reason, you should still be moving and trying to maintain control of your space while always making NOISE!

If you cannot run fast but do have time to distance yourself from a threatening person, use physical objects around you to put obstacles between you and the perpetrator. Do this using the nose-to-nose method (see page 123). Imagine you run around a parked car and they are on the other side. Keep your nose in line with their nose even from the other side of the car. Every time they move, keep your body in line with theirs but on the opposite side of the car, thus maintaining the distance between you. Do this in conjunction with making lots of noise. You can bang on the car (and maybe set off an alarm in the process), but keep your nose on their nose. This tactic can be used with a variety of other obstacles, such as bins, lampposts or bus stops. Parked cars are the ideal obstruction, though, as they are big enough to keep the perpetrator at bay, but small enough to run around quickly.

Always move in diagonal lines. This allows you to move out of the way less obviously, but with your nose still facing your opponent.

Running and then climbing onto a car can be a useful tactic if you have the time to do so. If the aggressor is hot on your tail, running to the side – of a nearby car or any large object you can get around quickly – is a better option as we do not want to turn our back on them. If you do climb onto a car this elevates you, and they would also have to climb on to get to you, which would alert others to your whereabouts. Regardless of what you opt to do, do not stop making noise.

Going underneath a large, parked vehicle is only possible if you are at quite a distance from the perpetrator and is most useful if you are looking to hide – in which case you should obviously not make any noise and alert the police using a silent call if you can (see Resources, page 228). If they were to try to pull you out, you could hold onto the bottom of the car. This tactic should be used as a final option, because while it hides you from the perpetrator, it also hides you from any onlookers, but it could still be helpful in certain situations.

<u>E</u>VERYTHING and anything can be your weapon!

'Make the most of what you have.'
FIGHTING PRINCIPLE

This principle I find very useful. It's the same tactic as using a parked car as an obstacle. If you are facing a very high-level threat, or the person trying to harm you is a lot bigger and stronger than you, using any object that might be to hand as a weapon can be an equaliser. You can use anything and everything around you to create time and space, to help you get away to safety. This could mean, for example, throwing something at their eyes to disrupt their vision. If necessary, you can follow up the throw with a strike; they are less likely to see it coming because you have disrupted their vision, and the strike may incapacitate them enough to make their response slower.

The best example of this tactic that I've seen is actually in Jackie Chan's fighting scenes. Although these are obviously choreographed movies, it's a very common and useful fighting principle. He will literally use any object to protect himself, and I always teach my students how to apply this tactic, as it's likely we will have something in our hands or nearby if we're ever attacked.

How to use everyday objects as survival weapons

If a threat is posed while you are holding an object, the best and most effective thing to do is to use what you have in your hand to help you, even if that's a magazine, book, water bottle or umbrella. You are most likely to be holding whatever it may be in your dominant hand, and it can take too long to let go of the object and use your hand, so instead of losing those precious seconds, just use whatever you're holding to your advantage. As a further upside, it often takes attackers by surprise.

THROWING OBJECTS

When throwing objects, the below principles must be kept in mind:

— Throw, strike or flick (depending on the object) 'from where your hands lie' – in other words, do not pull your hands back before initiating the throw. The same applies when striking. (See page 121.)

— Relax your arms and aim to send energy out, just as you would when throwing a ball.

A mobile phone

While you obviously would not want to damage your phone, it is the thing we're most likely to have to hand, and it is a great tool, particularly if you have a strong phone case. You can buy cases made for those who work on industrial sites – not only are they better protection for your phone, but if you did need to use your phone to stop someone hurting you then it's of much better use with a good case.

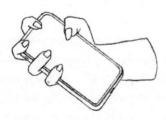

How to hold: Make sure one or two fingers are at the top of the phone to prevent it sliding with the strike. Have a firm and tight grip.

How to use: Strike with the edge of the phone at the weak points of the face: the bridge of the nose, the temple and the throat.

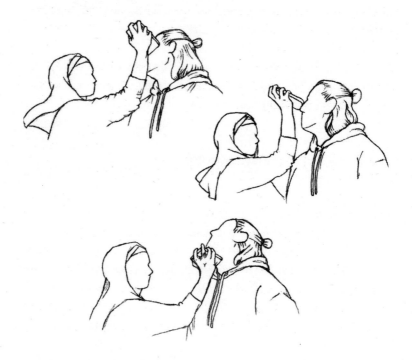

A bag

A small clutch bag can be thrown or held in your palm. Use it in the same way you would when you palm someone (see page 141). Keep the small bag in front of your hand and use it as a palm.

A larger bag can be thrown towards the legs of your aggressor as they run towards you, gaining you some time to run away. If you have the choice, however, avoid throwing anything that contains personal information.

Small blunt objects

This could be a car key, a pen or a small bottle of hairspray. The hairspray can be used as a legal alternative to pepper spray, or it can be held and used in a similar way to the other objects.

How to hold: Grip with your fingers curled around the object and your thumb supporting the top. The striking side of the hand is where the base of the object should be.

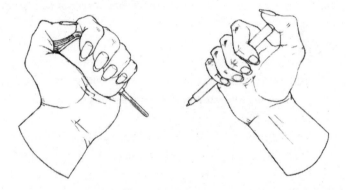

How to use: Imagine how you would use the side of your hand to chop. The blade of the hand is where the object will be used, e.g. palm facing up and striking down diagonally with the object, or palm facing down and striking down diagonally with the object.

If you have the object in your right hand and are striking the right side of your opponent (the right side of the face, right eye, right temple), use the object with your hand facing up and strike down diagonally. If you need to strike the left side with your right hand, you can turn your palm down and strike using the object this way, just like you would with an open-hand strike (see page 140). The same applies the other way round if striking with your left hand.

A heavy bunch of keys

It's actually not very practical to just hold a standard key in between your fingers unless it's a car key, which is a lot bigger and more stable. If you have a large bunch of keys, they will do more damage if you throw them at the person – just ensure that they aren't also your only means of safety, such as getting into your car. It is also important to ensure that the keys do not include any personal information.

A book

Books are chunky objects that can make effective weapons and can be particularly useful in a harassment situation on public transport, for example.

How to hold: Grasp firmly with the spine facing out, with the thumb on one side of the cover and the rest of your fingers on the other. If using a paperback, squeeze tightly to harden the spine.

How to use: Strike firmly with the spine. For example, if a person sits next to you on public transport and tries to put their arm around you:

1. Lock the perpetrator's leg by hooking your foot around their ankle and pushing their knee out with yours, then push out your closest arm at a 90-degree angle, holding the book in your other hand, spine out, ready to strike. Keep the book on your centre line.
2. If he tries to grab, strike his thumb with the book's spine. If he doesn't try to grab you, you can move on to Step 3.
3. Using the spine of the book, strike their nose or throat, or both, moving swiftly from your centre line.

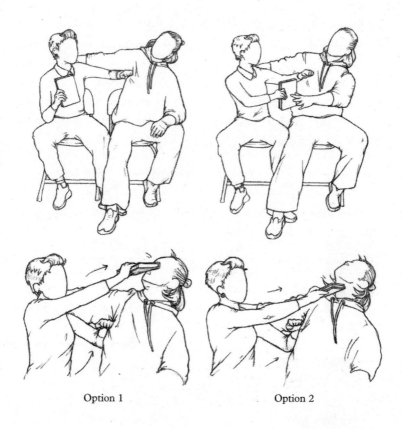

Option 1   Option 2

An umbrella, a bottle or a rolled-up newspaper or magazine
All of these everyday objects can effectively be used as a truncheon.

How to hold: Grip firmly around one end, or around the bottle neck.

How to use: There are various ways to strike with these objects:

a) Strike the perpetrator's attacking hand with the object.

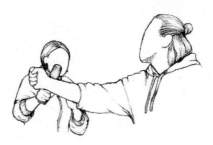

b) Grab their attacking arm with your free hand and strike a weak target using the chosen object.

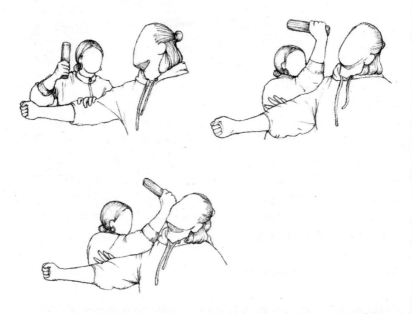

c) If they try to hit you using a circular strike, block the punch with your free arm, move into the open space and strike a weak target such as the nose, temple or throat with the base of your object. Aim for their centre line.

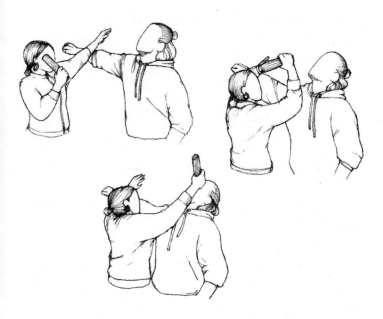

Window wipers

Window wipers are a great weapon if you have time to slide them off a car and know how – a whip across the face will keep the attacker away and in a lot of pain. Plus, using one requires no real strength or skill. Try to keep all strikes non-telegraphic, or with minimal movement; don't pull back to hit them as you will show them what you are about to do. Flick it like you would a towel. This makes the attack much harder to stop.

ATTACK the Weakest Targets

A good strike is not only about the end result, but also knowing how best to get there. Here is a checklist of what makes a good strike:

- Technique.
- Location – a weak target that requires minimum force.

- Strike frequency – keep your elbows behind your hands and your body behind your elbows: this maximises the energy exerted and is the difference between using just your hand's force and using a combination of hand, elbow and body force in one strike.
- Difficult to see coming (non-telegraphic).
- Simple and direct.

And there are several basic principles we can apply to ensure good results:

- Know your targets.
- Know your weapons.
- Use non-telegraphic moves.
- Use the shortest, most direct route to the target.
- Use economy of motion, i.e. generate maximum force with minimum effort.

There are so many strike techniques you can use, but I will list here what I feel are the simplest and easiest to execute, based on the four Distance Lines outlined earlier in the chapter (see page 116).

Distance Line 1 (legs)

The mechanics of a good kick is to lift from the knee. If you try to just lift your foot it will feel heavy, as if you are lifting your entire leg. Hinge everything from the knee instead.

It's useful to bear this in mind if you were to knee someone as well, because if they block it you can use your foot to kick a lower target. For example, I try to knee someone in the groin, the groin is blocked by their hand, so my foot hinges from my knee to kick their knee. After kicking, I don't leave my foot up or pull it back; I can step forward and use my other leg for another kick. When it comes to kicking, keep in mind that a knee can be a kick and a kick can be a step. Below are some strikes to try:

Whip kick/groin kick
A useful strike, particularly if your hands are incapacitated, that targets the sensitive groin area.

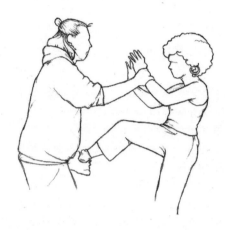

1. Point your toes down.
2. Use the top part of your foot, where you'd usually have laces.
3. Lift the knee to kick using a flick motion.

Diagonal stamp kick
Your primary target here is the person's knee. This strike is particularly useful if someone grabs your hands, hair, body or clothes. It takes little effort and can do a lot of damage. Your opponent will likely experience a break in focus due to pain or even feel incapacitated, leaving you able to break free and run.

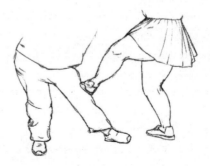

1. Lift your knee up and push down diagonally. Do not pull your leg back. The motion should be similar to stepping over a low hedge or gate.
2. Aim for the top of the opponent's knee joint or directly onto it.
3. Focus all your force through your heel. As this is not a push kick, imagine you have a stick leaning against a wall and you want to snap it in two with your foot.
4. This strike can also be used at Distance Lines 2 and 3, as just by lifting your knee higher you can stamp down and through, but it can also be used as close as six inches from your target. It's important to note when kicking someone's legs that you should keep your foot horizontal, so it is less likely to slide off their leg. The leg is a narrow target, so you're more likely to land a strike with a horizontal foot.

Distance Line 2 (hands, knees)

Open-hand strikes are some of my favourite weapons. They can allow you a longer reach, and become even more powerful the more relaxed you are.

Palm

There are several iterations of a palm strike, using different hand formations and motions, which can favour different targets. The basic technique, however, is the same for all of them:

1. To generate good power with a palm you should relax your arm, keeping your elbow low and bent behind and in line with the base of the palm.
2. Fire from the elbow using the base of the palm; this is the strongest point, as it's supported by your forearm bones.

Flat, open palm: Projected forward in a straight line, this can be used to strike key weak targets:

- the nose (directed upwards or downwards, depending on the opponent's position and whether they are taller or shorter than you)
- the chin (directed upwards, particularly if their mouth is open)
- ear (if the opponent has turned their head to the side)

Reverse palm: Projected upwards or downwards, this can be used to target:

- the groin. If you are bear hugged over both arms from the front or behind but your forearms are still free to move, move your hips to one side and use your palm to strike the groin.
- the nose. This is done by lifting the palm up towards opponent's nose when they are in a bent-over or horizontal position – for example, if they lunge at your legs to try to grab them.

Side palm: Much more powerful than a slap, because of the elbow position lined up behind the base of the palm, the side-palm strike is useful for targeting:

- the jaw
- ears (with cupped palm)

Blade of the hand

The highlighted area below is what we call the blade of the hand. This area can be used for the same targets whether the blade of the hand is facing down or up. When facing up it looks similar to side palm, but you would use the bladed area to chop. It's important to note that your fingers should be kept together for this motion.

The main targets for the blade of the hand are:
- the nose
- the throat (front and side)

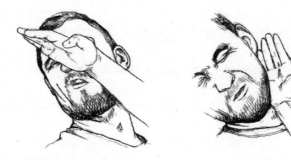

Punch

It took me a long time to generate the power and learn the technique of a punch. I often damaged my wrist as I didn't know how to protect it when striking heavy bags or hard targets. When using a fist for self-defence without sufficient training, it's better to strike really soft targets (like the throat).

How to make a fist:
1. Fold your fingers first.
2. Fold your thumb on the outside, hugging the second joint of the fingers.
3. Make the striking part of the fist look like a rectangular box.
4. Keep the fist in line with the wrist and the bones of your forearm.

CHAIN STRIKES

Chain strikes are some of the most difficult to defend against due to their rapid-fire nature. The best way to deliver chain strikes is in straight lines along the shortest route, which means you won't need to pull back at any point. A chain strike automatically resets one hand as the other is in action, maintaining the best defence position of having one hand forward as the other is further back gaining momentum. It has been estimated that on average chain strikes can deliver 8–11 strikes per second. This is the difference between trying to dodge an arrow or a machine gun firing arrows. A chain strike can be carried out with any straight-line moves, including chain palms and chain punches.

The reason this is so useful is that if one of our strikes is not enough against a larger opponent, it takes just one second to fire numerous strikes to the same area and to more than one target as the aggressor moves about. If someone is advancing and you strike their nose with one or two of the strikes, their head is likely to pull back, and you can proceed to strike the ear or throat, depending on how they move, with the rest of the strikes in your chain.

We call this bouncing from one target to another. It's very effective because as the person's focus is drawn to your first strike, you're already moving on to another.

Double punch: Aimed at soft targets, this is one of the most powerful strikes and one of the most difficult to defend. It's useful when an opponent opens up their centre and for sending someone back a significant distance in order to escape. Just ensure your elbows are low and in front of your own ribs so that when you step with the strike your body weight can be used to generate further force.

A double punch can target two soft areas at once, such as:

- the nose and throat
- the throat and solar plexus (pictured)

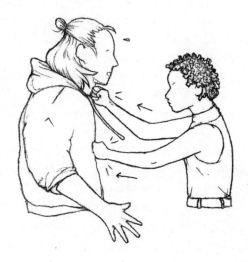

Eye strike using the thumb: I've found this easier and more effective than straight finger attacks, particularly when I was a beginner. I would still go to this rather than finger strikes – it's safer for you and more effective. There is a saying to help with the application – you 'stroke the face and take the eye', pushing the thumb into the eye socket. Any strike that prompts someone's natural instinct to focus on themselves – so ones that disrupt sight and airways – is great.

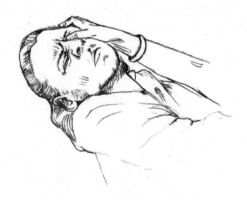

Knees

The best way to knee is in a straight line. Point your toes down when you knee, as it makes the move sharper and faster than when your foot is flat and parallel to the floor.

Distance Line 3 (elbows)

Front of elbows

When using the front of the elbow, keep your hand open. Strike with the part that is towards the top of your forearm and closest to the elbow point – about a fist's width is the area you should use. The reason we leave our hand open is because it allows the force to fly out more. If you close your fist, then try to strike with the front of your elbow; you will feel some restriction in its delivery, but if you open it you are able to send out more energy.

Horizontal elbow strike: Hold your arm in a horizontal position in front of your body with your hand open, then strike with the front part of your elbow. Try to keep your elbow in line with your hips so you can turn your body in conjunction with the elbow's movement, thus creating more force in the strike.

Your main targets for this move are:

- the jaw
- the temple
- the throat
- the nose

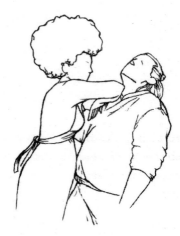

Diagonal downward elbow strike: Use the same action as the horizontal strike, but lift your elbow slightly, then strike down on the same targets using a diagonal line. This is useful to strike facial targets on taller attackers.

Back of elbows

More commonly used against attackers who come from behind, the back part of the elbow is again an area around a fist's width from the point of the elbow to the back of your upper arm. When using this side of your elbow close your fists – you can generate more force when striking and the closing muscles protect the nerves at the back of your elbow at same time.

Vertical downward elbow strike: Hold your arm vertically in front of your body, with your fist up at 12 o'clock and your elbow down at 6 o'clock. Bring down the back of the elbow onto the target. This is commonly used when the attacker is horizontal; for example, if they are bending down to grab your legs, you have sent their head back with a strike or they have grabbed your hair and you are striking their bicep.

Targets can include:

- the back of the head
- the back of the neck
- the spine

Vertical backward elbow strike: Keeping your arm vertical in line with your body, jab the back of the elbow backwards to the target. This move is commonly used against attacks from behind.

Likely targets, depending on the attacker's position, are:

- the ribs
- the groin

Horizontal backward elbow strike: Just like the horizontal front-elbow strike above: your arm is in the same position, but your fist is closed and you are striking backwards with the back of the elbow.

Distance Line 4 (body)

Distance 4 is body to body, or when you need to use your body to move out of the way of an oncoming attack. This could be when someone is very close, maybe grabbing your body from behind or from the front over the arms, or when someone is advancing with an attack so that you need to turn your body as well as deflect with your hands.

The weapons you can use at the body-to-body distance are:

Reverse palm: If someone grabs your body from behind and over your arms, you are still able to move your forearms and also your hips. To execute this strike, move your hips to the side and throw your palm backwards to groin area.

Wrist strike: This move is described as 'lifting the tea bag from the cup' and can be used when someone grabs your body from the front over your arms. In this situation your hands and forearms can move. To execute this move, swing your wrist forward to the groin; the hand position will be as if you are lifting a tea bag from the cup. The wrist flies forward to the groin.

Shoulder strike: If someone tries to grab your body from the side, you can step in and butt them with your shoulder. This is utilised at the last minute before the arms link around you and can be used from up to an inch's distance from their body to your shoulder. Simply step sideways like a crab between their legs, attacking and striking their sternum or solar plexus with your shoulder joint. This should be a big step, keeping your head in line with your spine as you do so.

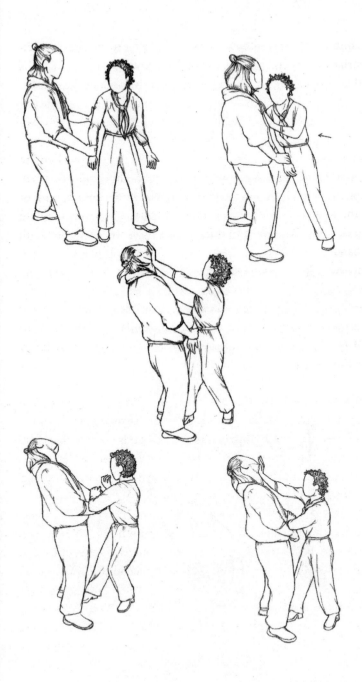

Leg locks: When someone is body to body, be it grabbing you from the side, front or back, or sitting really close to you, you can use their proximity to your advantage by combining arm strikes and defensive techniques with leg locks. The leg lock weakens both their ankle and the knee, while controlling their head at the same time destabilises them.

Leg lock from the side: Hook your foot around the inside of their foot, slotting it as close to theirs as possible, then with the same leg circle your knee around the outside of their knee so your foot is on the inside of their ankle and then use your knee as a lever, crushing the outside of their knee while keeping their ankle hooked. This can be used if someone tries to grab you or hold you side-on, like putting their arm around you or standing next to you to get you in a headlock, or sitting too close to you on a bench or public transport and trying to touch you. Use this to control their lower body, which will help you control their upper body.

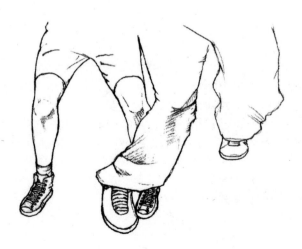

Leg lock from behind: This lock is used when we are grabbed from behind or lifted. Hook your leg on the inside of either of their legs (whichever you feel is closer) if you are being lifted; this will anchor yourself so it's difficult for someone to move you and will likely result in them falling over.

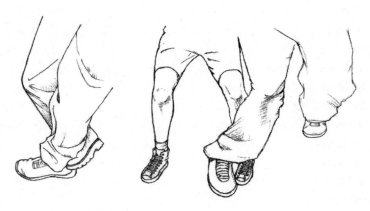

If lifted   If grabbed from behind but not lifted

CALL for Help

Calling for help is not only a tactic for stopping an attack; it should continue after an attack as well. Even if the attack was merely an attempt and you managed to get away, as soon as you are able to leave the situation **CALL** someone for help, be that the police or family. Go somewhere you can find help and make lots of noise on your way. It's natural to feel shaken and to want to just go home right away, but for your safety it's vital that you get the help and support you need immediately.

<u>T</u>ELL Someone

Remember, it is important to tell someone what happened sooner rather than later, when it's still fresh in your mind and you can better remember the important details. You can record a voice note while waiting for help to arrive, or relay the incident to an operator when calling for assistance.

9.

GATES AND ANGLES
(IMMINENT DANGER: PART 2)

This chapter will introduce ways to defend yourself against attacks coming from the most common angles and aimed at the most common areas of the body (known as 'gates'), and even how to deal with attempted touches, grabs or slaps before they can reach you. For me, developing these skills was not only about practice, experience and learning an automatic defensive reflex; it was also about understanding the science behind them – I learned how to generate enough counterstrike force from my body, how to move and evade attacks in the most subtle way, the best shapes or positions I needed to create with my limbs to deflect attacks without needing a greater force, how to do that with an attack from any angle to any area of my body and lastly, how to use the attacker's momentum and movement to my advantage and their disadvantage.

Because the moves, principles and defences are born from an understanding of physics and geometry, they can deflect a stronger opposing force from a potentially larger attacker efficiently, using minimal energy. This knowledge gave me faith that the oncoming blows were dependable, predictable, and if I just stuck to the correct lines and shapes, I could deflect them and strike back all at once.

In this chapter we will look at the best methods for developing

these skills, while tying in the principles we have been using throughout this book. You will learn that developing a reaction to deflect a
person's hands from early on will also give you the chance to prevent
them getting any closer, and give you an adaptable skill that can be
tailored to the level of threat you face. For example, if someone wants
to grab your hair, but you have a reaction to protect that area and
know how to move when an attack comes from that angle, that person
can't get to your hair so easily. This can be used in lower-level-threat
scenarios of setting physical boundaries, too. Maybe someone says,
'I like your necklace', and then tries to touch your necklace and you
are not comfortable with this; you can use your limbs to deflect their
hand in a subtle way that is proportionate to the situation and sets a
boundary. But the good news is the techniques remain the same even
if the threat is higher. The only difference is the severity and force
used, and determining if you need to add a counterstrike.

This will depend on your assessment of the situation. If it's a
physical-boundary violation like touching your necklace or hair
but the threat may not be considered high then you can simply use
the defence minus the strike, and with little dynamic force. In this
instance, it could be dealt with by just using a deflective move along
with a verbal boundary, such as, 'Use words, not hands.' If it's a
touch that falls under sexual assault, the level of threat is higher, so
you may need to combine the deflective move with a counterstrike,
and you may need to move if they are advancing and dominating
your space, all at a faster pace and with more force. But it's the same
move; just matching the speed and momentum of the attacker. If
the attack on these angles is a strike then the same moves are used,
but the skill required to execute them needs training, and it would
be irresponsible of me to suggest otherwise. Strike defence skill
requires much more training because this type of attack is faster and
stronger, and the attacker is likely to be more mobile – and it is not
easy to hit a moving target. This book and this chapter are intended
to give you the starting tools on this journey, but in truth there are

many areas of self-defence that are advanced and require assistance for development.

ESSENTIAL SKILLS

The skills needed to be sufficient in defending against strikes to all areas of the body (which we separate into 'gates') and coming from all angles are:

- A very good ability to detect the distance between you and your opponent.
- A very good knowledge of your range as well as how to learn your opponent's range. This includes: how to use your distance lines of defence instinctively (if they are within kicking range, punching/knee range, elbow range, etc.) and how to use your limbs at those ranges to defend oncoming blows, and how to move your head if they get past all these lines of defence and are about to land a strike.
- The ability to respond to different speeds.
- The ability to adapt if they change angle and target suddenly.
- The ability to adapt to tricks and feints.
- Very good strike accuracy on a moving target.
- Tactics on how to bring the head down if your attacker is too tall.
- Good speed, agility, striking force and reflexes.

The moves and principles used to deflect strikes from any angles are the same for any advance or attack, so this chapter will cover the foundations of developing these defence skills, with the focus on those kinds of attacks that move more slowly towards you (a touch, grab, push, etc.), as they are both more common and much more useful to learn about at this stage. It will also give examples of how you can develop these moves into sufficient strike defence skills if the advances progress to a higher level of threat.

What makes a good deflecting move?

An effective deflecting move:
- is simple and easy to apply.
- is easily adaptable from strike to defence and vice versa.
- redirects a force instead of trying to stop or block it.
- doesn't require strength for it to be effective.
- enables you to strike back simultaneously if needed.
- can be adapted to any level of threat.

Below I will explore the principles that make a good strike defence possible.

THE SCIENCE OF DEFENCE

There are three scientific principles that underpin the dynamics of an effective defence:

1. Trying to stop a force in motion that is greater than our own is not possible, so we must use the laws of physics to allow it to continue but pass us by. We can do this by either not being on the intended path (by moving or turning) or by redirecting the oncoming force. When it comes to deflecting an attack efficiently, it's all about the shapes and motion we create with our hands. Using a static blocking move is no good if the force that is

coming in is greater than our own, so instead we want to create a motion that encourages an oncoming force to be redirected without trying to stop it or move it away from its target. A wedge-shaped defence (see page 124) that travels forward to intercept an oncoming attack would easily and efficiently redirect the opponent's force.

2. To develop enough force in our counterstrikes we must understand that force is the product of mass and acceleration. With a strong body structure, we can use the mass behind our strikes (our body) to generate more force. Firing from a low elbow position allows us the acceleration to generate enough force while still maintaining a good structure behind it, and this also means we do not have to pull our hands back before striking. This allows us to be non-telegraphic and to use the shortest line of attack in our moves. By knowing the structure of our defences and using theories like nose to nose (see page 123) we can also borrow our opponent's force, which adds to our own.

3. Every action has an opposite and equal reaction, and this can be utilised to borrow your opponent's force without having to overcome it. Think of your body structure like a revolving door. When you push the door away on the right side, the left side moves forward. Using the vertical mid-centre line of our body as a reference, we can see where our left side and right side are divided, and also where our centre is. This allows us to use our body in a similar fashion to the revolving door. Imagine someone pushes your right shoulder; with good structure, positioning and grounding, you can turn your body without losing balance. Without them, you can be knocked off balance. A good defence

will use the hands to detect how great the force is, so the body will then know when to turn, and in which direction. Understanding the different zones of your body and how they can respond to attack will help you take advantage of that force.

THE EIGHT GATES THEORY

One of the most revolutionary theories in self-defence in my opinion is the 'eight gates theory'. This is used as a method to train and understand how to manage attacks coming from different angles to different parts of the body. The application and understanding of it allows you to compartmentalise your repertoire of defences according to each area, or gate, of the body. This makes the decision on how to defend yourself a lot simpler. An attack to a specific area can only happen in certain ways and therefore has certain responses that belong to it.

After practising the defences to all the gates coming from different angles, you will start to develop automatic responses, which will allow you to react to an attack to any area before conscious thought. This is so useful if you are surprised or prone to freezing, as it allows your hands to move instinctively and can, over time, literally rewrite your nervous system, as if programming the moves into your arms.

To distinguish the eight gates, we draw a vertical midline through the body. We make another line across the centre point horizontally (in line with the solar plexus). At the lowest point that we can defend with our hands, which is where our wrists lie (in line with the groin), we draw another horizontal line across the body. And another is drawn across the knees. This divides the upper and lower body into four quarters each, so as you can see in the diagram below, there are eight gates in total, separated into the lower, middle and upper gates, and the left side and right side.

Right and left are laid out from the defender's perspective, so gates 1, 3, 5 and 7 are all on the right side of your body, and gates 2, 4, 6 and 8 are on the left side. The left hand is primarily used at the beginner stages to defend the left side, and the right hand to defend the right, while the other is responsible for a counterstrike if needed. If the attack is closer to the centre, you can choose which hand to use. For example, if someone tries to touch your face using their right hand in a straight line, you could defend this by using your left or right hand because it is at the centre. You can also choose to position yourself on the outside of the limb they are attacking with, rather than the inside; this is safer because you are further away from both their hands – for example, deflecting their attack to your right side and, if needed, turning your right side away allows you to be on the outside of their arm, not on the inside. This is much harder to do with circular or rounds moves coming in from a wide position, when you are usually on the inside of their attacking limb and must defend with your hands on the inside, as this is the shortest route to the attack.

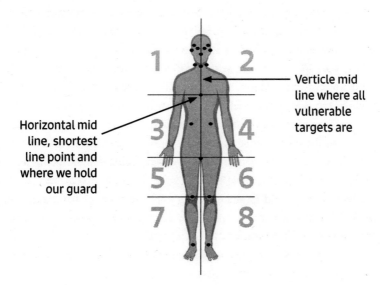

Verticle mid line where all vulnerable targets are

Horizontal mid line, shortest line point and where we hold our guard

A good defence system will always have control of their opponent's three levels (upper, middle and low) at the same time. When you first start learning you should train each gate individually but repetitively. The idea is that your hands always try to maintain two lines of defence in the guard position by having one forward and one back, but you do not have to stick to that position. As mentioned, ideally we want to use our left hand to defend the attacks on our left side and our right hand to counter at the same time, and vice versa. But we need to be as adaptable as possible, so you can swap them around – both hands should be trained independently to move at the same time.

Because you have two hands at different distances, if the front hand fails, the rear hand can take over. You can change your hand positions at any time; they are both already in position to either defend or attack. For example, if a circular or round attack was coming in wide on my upper left side – gate 2 – and my right hand was forward, it would be better to use my left hand to defend it as that is closer to the attack; if I used my right hand to defend an attack on my left, I would be exposed to a second attack from my opponent's left side and neither of my hands would be near enough to defend it.

This skill does require training for efficiency and understanding, but once you've developed good reactions and reflexes in the upper gates, you can move on to practise defending the lower gates using the same concepts. When you're familiar with this method, you're prepared to defend yourself against a variety of attacks.

The stage of development with the eight-gates method is that you first learn the defences of the upper gates (1, 2, 3 and 4, and along the centre line, high, medium and low) and once you are proficient in singular defences of one specific gate from all angels, you then change the gates and angles randomly. The next stage is to learn to defend against more than one attack at a time to the same gate or to different gates. Then you would practise the defences with an added counterstrike with either a step in or a turn. Once proficient, you can practise this at different distances to learn your range and the range of your opponent. Then it's a case of adding speed, power and more advanced attacks. Once the upper gates are mastered, you can start using the same method to develop your defences of the lower gates. This is how the eight gates theory can help you develop the knowledge and skills to manage attacks from all angles, to all areas and at all levels of threat.

BE DYNAMIC AND ACTIVE IN YOUR EXECUTION

The first rule of good defence is that you must be active with your moves. You will always be quicker off the mark with your defences if you are dynamic and active in your execution instead of passive. Let's imagine the game 'whack a mole', where your aim is to strike the moles' heads as soon as they pop up. The reason you can react quickly in this game is because you are being active. Similarly, your defending hand will move much faster if you react actively, almost as if your moves are trying to attack your opponent's arms. If your aim is simply to defend, you'll always be slower. It's about being offensive rather than just defensive. Ideally, we should be meeting the strike instead of waiting for it, which enables us to intercept it earlier and deflect it sooner.

Use the shortest-line principle

Using the shortest-line principle will always help you to choose the quickest and most direct path of defence and counterattack. Projecting out from the intersecting point of the horizontal and vertical mid-lines is the body's three-dimensional centre line. If you trace this line to your opponent's centre-line point, this creates the shortest, most direct route between you, and it is where we hold our pre-fight guard position (creating two lines of defence with our hands).

If the line of the attack is close to this centre point, you can choose to defend on the outside of their attack, placing yourself on one side of both of their arms, which is the best position to be in. But if they use circular or round strikes and you are in closer proximity, the shortest route would be for you to defend on the inside of that strike by stepping forward and invading their stance completely. This is using the shortest-line principle.

For example, if your opponent comes in with a straight attack to your centre, you cannot occupy the same space, so you must let the force go past you. By using your hands to create a wedge shape and projecting forward in this shape, making the move three-dimensional, it intercepts the oncoming limb and redirects its force, and will also help you feel if you need to turn. Remember that for straight attacks to the centre, you can choose which hand you use to defend and strike.

If they were to use a circular angled strike instead, as in the illustration below, they are not occupying the centre; they are taking a longer route, so you can leave later and still arrive first by using a straight-line defence and counter – the shortest and quickest line of attack. Just ensure you step inside the attack circle, still using a wedge shape to defend, and strike at the same time with your other hand. If they attack your upper-left gate with a circular attack, use your left hand to defend, step in towards them and strike a weak target with your right hand.

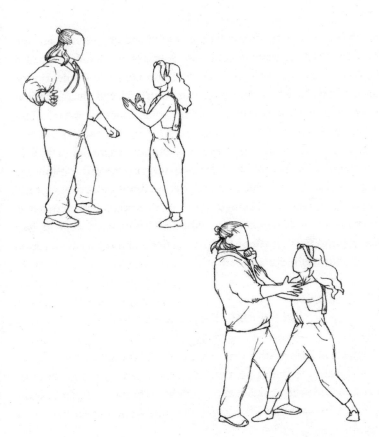

Use wedge theory to anticipate an attack

As mentioned in Chapter 8: Strategies and Tactics, wedge theory allows you to create a wedge shape with your body in order to efficiently defend attacks. This three-dimensional defence principle is the best way to detect how to deflect an oncoming strike. By moving your hands toward their hands – we call this 'bridging forward' – you can meet the attack along its path, intercept it and better determine how to redirect it. The point of contact would be their forearm; the area roughly a fist's distance from the point where the hand ends and the forearm starts. You use the same part of your forearm to connect too. Once you have touch you have a second pair of eyes and can feel how they move as well as see. This is useful if they suddenly change attack or direction, or if the lighting is low. On the flip side, if you wait for their strike to arrive, you are static and will always have a slower, more reactionary response.

This is the difference between using your arms to block an attack or using them to deflect it. If you try to predict where the strike will land and block it, you will have to solely rely on strength and timing, but if you use this principle, you're meeting them on their path, with a deflecting move. So although we use our distance lines of defence (see page 116) to help us know when and how to move, it is still important to meet the force with our hands. It allows us to be active and dynamic in our execution.

LET'S PUT IT ALL TOGETHER

Now we will look at how we can defend the upper four gates (1, 2, 3 and 4, and the centre points), first against straight or linear lines of attack, and then against circular angles, tying in the fighting principles we've looked at. First, here is a reminder of the main defence principles:

— Use the shortest, most direct route of defence and attack (move from your centre line to meet the attack).
— Move from where your hands lie so you do not telegraph your defence (i.e. don't pull your hands back before you move them); even if your hands are down when you need to defend, just move them from that position to the centre line to execute the defence or attack.
— Be three-dimensional in your defence using forward motions and wedge-shaped postures, as opposed to blocking or trying to use horizontal defences to force the

attack across your body.
— When there is a need to counterattack (when the level of threat is high) defend and attack at the same time. Remember, the targets closer to the centre of the body are the weakest.
— Use your four distance lines of defence (see page 116): if you need to counterstrike, use the strikes that are available to you (if your opponent is within kicking range then kick; if within hand and knee range then strike with hands or knees, etc. If they are advancing in past your first three distance lines then you need to turn).
— With a very high-level threat make the most of what you have (if you have an everyday object in your hand that can be used as a weapon, then use that to counter).

Straight or linear advance to the centre or upper gates

Below are some options if a person is advancing to attack the upper centre of your body (for example, to grab your chest, touch your face or neck, or grab your throat).

Option 1

The first option we can use is a movement known as 'slapping hand', which is like a cat's paw. This movement uses the palm of the hand as though you are aiming to slap the part of their forearm near the wrist. It can be used if a person is trying to advance to your centre line or inside your front hand in a fast but not particularly heavy motion. Imagine someone is trying to snatch your necklace or poke you in the chest – the 'slapping hand' can be used here, but the direction of our hand is important. Don't swat away across your body; instead, move in a forward motion, meeting your opponent's hand on the route it is travelling. This is a more effective way to deflect the oncoming force.

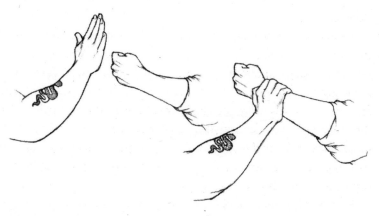

Option 2

We can also use a movement known as 'bridging arm', which means holding your arm in a position that looks like a snake. Turn your hand over so your palm is facing the floor and use the outside of your forearm to intercept the outside of your opponent's arm. By advancing your hand forward and creating a wedge shape, you can grab their arm with more control, in a snap-like motion to the side.

If the threat isn't high, you will not need to counter. Just set a verbal boundary along with the defensive move. But if it is an attack, sexual assault (trying to grab your chest, for example) or higher threat, you can counterattack by palming their ear with your other hand at the same time as you intercept their forearm. Because you are turning their body slightly as you intercept their forearm, the ear is exposed and therefore a good target.

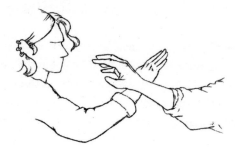

Option 3

If the person is advancing, dominating the centre line and closing the distance between you, you could use the wedged 'bridging arm' position to defend, but you could also turn your gates. Just like a revolving door, as one side goes back, the other side goes forward; the side that turns away uses the wedge-shaped defence move and the other side uses a counterattack. This allows the attacker's force to advance even further, creating more impact when we land our strike because they are moving towards it, and yet their target has turned away and is no longer there.

To turn, pivot the foot you are taking away from the attack, while keeping the other foot planted. If your opponent is very big, you can use the falling leaf step (see page 115) to allow you to step and turn at the same time.

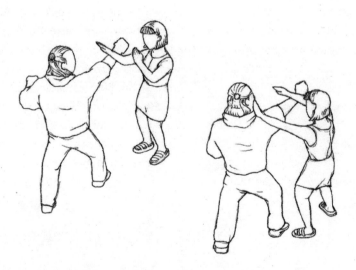

Straight or linear advance towards the mid-centre or lower gates

Below are some options if a person is advancing with a move aimed at your lower gates or mid-centre points (for example, to touch or grab your abdomen, waist or groin).

Option 1

This movement is known as 'splitting hand' and it's like a chop down towards an oncoming limb. If someone tries to grab or touch your groin area, or if they were to try to strike the low-centre point of your tummy, throw your hand down to the outside of their forearm using a cutting motion, meeting them at your centre line. (Remember that strikes are faster than grabs or touches and use more force so it would require training to develop the technique for those.) If they advance in, you can turn as in Option 3 of the upper or central attacks above. And if you realise they are trying to touch your groin area and the threat is higher, a counterstrike to the ear drum, nose or eye can give you time to escape.

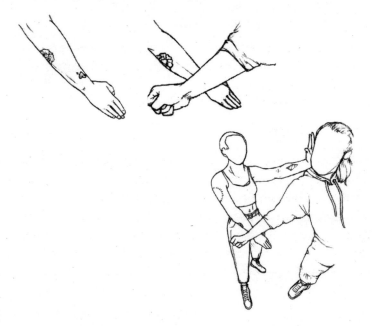

Option 2

Here we could also use the cat-paw 'slapping hand' move again. This technique is useful for defending against an advance travelling from a low hand position to a central area of the body. As before, use the palm of the hand as though you are aiming to slap the part of their forearm near the wrist. It's a fast move and can be used against a fast advance.

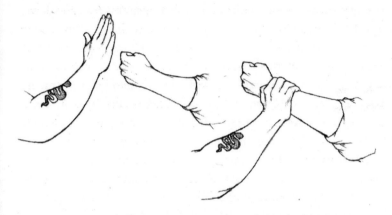

Wide or circular advance to the upper gates

Below are some options if a person advances towards or attacks your upper gates (gates 1 and 2) from a wide angle. They may be trying to touch the side of your face, grab your hair from the side or slap your face using a circular or round movement.

Option 1

If someone is violating your space but isn't a high-level threat, here you can use the 'bridging arm' technique again but on the inside of their arm this time (see page 166), creating a wedge shape as you move towards the person to intercept and deflect the advance. You can also set a verbal boundary (remember that if you are not comfortable with a person touching you then it is important you set that boundary), though a counterstrike won't be necessary.

Option 2

If the threat level is higher, such as a circular slap, strike or hair grab, and they move their hand but do not turn their body, you can follow up the bridging arm technique with a step in and a strike, such as an open vertical palm to the nose, so you are defending and attacking at the same time. Remember to be non-telegraphic in your moves and use straight-line attacks directly from your centre line. Your shortest route to defend is along the straight line so in this instance we can go on the inside.

Option 3

If the person slaps or grabs you with a heavier motion, turning their body as they do so, you can use the bridging arm to deflect their arm, and flow into the empty space as they are turning so you can stay nose to nose with them. Combine with a counterstrike to a weak target such as their eyes, nose, throat or ears. To do this, you should step inside of their hand movement (especially if it is a slap) because then you are no longer in the path of the circular attack, you are inside it. The timing of your defence and simultaneous counter-attack should be on the pull-back or rise of their arm. This allows you to unbalance them as their rotate, making it easier for you to use their force against them. So attack on their attack, rather than defending it and then countering, which would allow them time to regain stability and attack again.

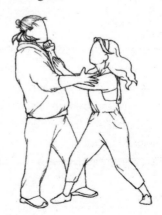

Option 4

As a last-minute defence of the upper gates against a circular attack if you are caught off-guard, are late with your reaction or your opponent moves more quickly than expected, you can use your upper arm to cover the targeted area – for example, if someone tries to slap or strike your face or grab your hair from the side, the area to cover would be the side of your head.

To execute this move you need to lift your elbow vertically, close to your head, as if aiming to touch your back with your hand. As you do this, dip your chin slightly and step in towards your attacker with a counterstrike to a weak target if needed, such as a punch to their throat.

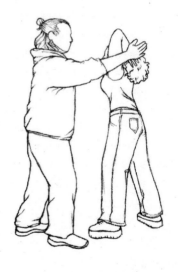
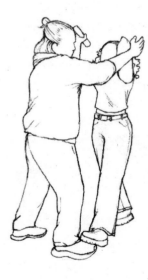

Wide or circular advances to the lower gates

Below are some options to defend wider or circular advances to your lower gates (gates 3 and 4), perhaps against someone who is standing in front of you but tries to grab or slap your bum from the side, or if they are already to your side and you notice they are about to grab or slap you.

Option 1

When the threat level is low, we can use a similar move to the 'splitting hand' technique to defend central mid-level advances. The move is practically the same – a chop downwards to deflect the advancing limb – but the end point is on your shoulder line rather than your centre.

Option 2

If the threat level is higher, you can use this move in the same way as the other defensive techniques by combining it with a strike, a step in and strike, or a step in and strike using nose to nose if your opponent turns. As this is a wide or circular attack, as before you should defend on the inside with this technique.

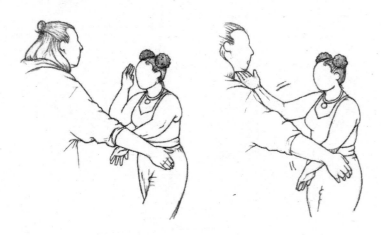

If you need to counterstrike a weak target in combination with any of these defences, the best weapons to use are:

— Open-hand vertical palm to the nose (see page 140).
— Side-palm strike to the throat using the blade of the hand (see page 142).
— Eye strike (see page 145).
— Punch to the throat.
— If your opponent's head is turned, a palm strike to the ear.

You can use chain strikes to any of these targets (see page 143).

10.

CONTROLLING ATTACKERS
(IMMINENT DANGER: PART 3)

GRABS, HOLDS, PINS AND CHOKES

Grabbing, holding, pinning and choking are the most common types of attack that violent people use against smaller people, and the most common attacks used against women. This is likely to be because the perpetrator's motivation is power; they want their target to feel powerless, so they carry out attacks that show their strength. That's not to say they never strike, but strikes are often combined with some form of grab.

To effectively deal with these sorts of attacks when your attacker is stronger than you, you cannot use your strength against their strength. You must use other means to overpower them, which is a skill that can be adapted to all areas of self-defence. In this chapter we will look at how to defend against someone who tries to physically control you in these ways.

If you are truly to overcome the urge to fight strength with strength, you need to be able to completely relax the area the person is trying to control so they do not feel any resistance. Doing so means there is no further attention given to the area, because they feel they have full control there, and this allows you to use other limbs and techniques they will not see coming.

These techniques and principles do not try to move, stop or

interrupt the perpetrator's action, but to keep them where they are already determined to be, so they only notice that you have moved when it's too late. Whatever they do, you can use it to your own advantage.

However, this is not an easy task – not because the techniques themselves are complex, but because we have to retrain our response not to fight strength with strength. Trying to wrestle the person away feels like the most natural response because you just want them off you. But there are other ways, which are not only natural, but also allow us to use economy of motion, rather than fighting to exhaustion to no avail. We can use *their* strength to *our* advantage, by not disrupting their action in the way they expect.

Some of these attacks may not seem that dangerous at first glance, but the feeling of being grabbed can trigger a shock in the body and will let you know the strength of your attacker. If they are restricting your airways, this is extremely high risk. If they are dragging you to an isolated area or vehicle, this is also extremely high risk. These would be Threat Level 5 attacks.

I know from my own experience that feeling the squeeze of someone who is a lot bigger and stronger than you messes with you psychologically; it can cause your entire body to go tense, even if they are just grabbing one wrist. It can seem as though you have already lost when you feel how strong they are, making it seem pointless to fight back. This is exactly why I take it very seriously if someone grabs my hand or blocks my way: it is not respectful behaviour.

Although it is not uncommon to freeze or feel powerless because someone has grabbed you and you feel their strength, I found that once I knew a way to respond that I could trust and rely on, a way that would make that unwanted action work in my favour, I stopped feeling powerless. Knowing how and where you *are* powerful is what matters, and if you don't know that then the negative is all you see. Knowledge truly is power and in this area of self-defence we will look at a variety of ways that you are powerful, how to use what is available to you and not concentrate on the unavailable, and how to keep your attacker's focus on where they think their power lies, so they won't see what you can do coming.

Any of the techniques shown in this chapter can be assigned to any level of threat. If it's low level, you can just use the disengaging or breaking-away techniques without the strike. Adding the strikes is for managing a higher level of threat; they help disrupt the thoughts of the attacker because instinctively we draw our attention to where we feel pain, so it's easier to *then* disengage and get away.

The acronym **GRABS** will help you remember what to do if you are being physically grabbed or controlled:

GIVE them what they want, just not how they want it.
REALISE what you do have and relax what you don't have.
ATTACK the weak points.
BREAKING POINTS – grip weaknesses.
SHORTEST LINE – if they go out, you go in. If they go in, you go out.

Now let's break down each stage of that acronym.

GIVE them what they want, just not how they want it

This principle is about controlling the situation through adaptation – swimming with the current, instead of against it. It literally changes the game as it cleverly illustrates that you do not need to fight your opponent's force with your force; instead, you borrow their force, which they have already given you, and use it to your advantage.

If executed correctly, this tactic is like a rope tied to a rock they are pulling at. All they are focused on is the rock. They are tugging away, but then the rope snaps and smacks them in the face. This can act as a psychological trick on the attacker, because it is unexpected and you are effectively boomeranging off their action and the direction their force is already going in.

Below are two examples of how to make the most of what you have in a single-grab scenario – they demonstrate the same grab to the wrist, but using two different directions of force:

1. They pull you in by the wrist – instead of pulling away from them, catapult yourself forward using their strength (which increases your acceleration and the power of your strikes) and palm a weak target, such as their chin (hitting upwards) or their nose, with your free hand using the shortest line of attack (see page 184).

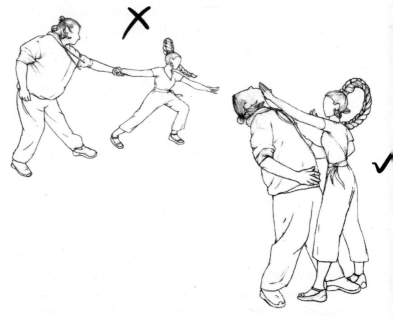

Striking with whatever you have free is very simple, and often comes as a surprise to the attacker. If someone grabs one hand and you are within Distance

Line 2 (hand-strike distance), strike with your free hand immediately and then disengage as described below. If you are within Distance Line 1 (kicking distance) when they grab (they may have much longer limbs than you), you can kick followed straight away by a hand strike, then disengage and exit. For example, a combination such as a stamp kick to the knee (see page 139) or a whip kick to the groin (see page 139) followed by a palm to the nose (see page 141) or an eye strike (see page 145) is great because the kicks encourage the attacker to instinctively bend, bringing their head closer in line with a direct strike.

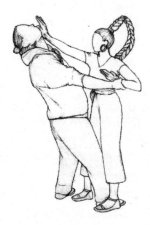

As soon as you have palmed their weak target, take your palming hand and, using the dynamic force disengaging technique (see page 125), slap it straight onto the wrist of the attacker's grabbing hand and at the same time pull your grabbed wrist out from between the thumb and fingers towards the centre of your own body.

The force of slapping and pulling at the same time makes this releasing technique more efficient. But the strike from the palm first is very important, as the opponent's head will go back and this will weaken their grip as well as break their focus. By going with the force rather than against it, you have been able to use your opponent's strength as well as your own.

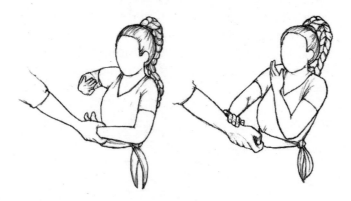

2. They push you back or walk towards you with a grab to the wrist. Because this is a grab to the left hand, the pressure when they walk in will be felt on that side, so as they come in turn your right side towards them and pull your left side back, like a revolving door. This allows their force to continue on its intended path.

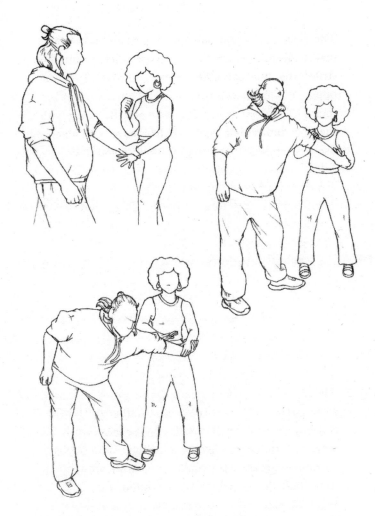

Use the beggar's palm position (see page 102) to weaken their grip and make it easier to either free your wrist or grab their wrist back in one smooth motion.

As you turn you can also strike a weak target with your free hand, e.g. palm their ear, stamp kick their knee or strike with your elbow while pulling their wrist up (see Chapter 8: Strategies and Tactics). To push your opponent down apply pressure on their elbow and lift their wrist up at the same time. Keep your own head up straight as you do this.

These techniques can both be used in parallel or diagonal positions. If parallel, you use disengagement techniques on the inside of their wrist; if diagonal, on the outside of the wrist. It's important to recognise that these are both the same grab; it's the direction of force that determines what we do in response. This is how we use their force against them.

<u>R</u>EALISE what you do have and relax what you don't have

The ability to realise what you DO have and not focus on what you DON'T have allows you to access the best ways to release yourself from your attacker's control in the most efficient way. We can do this even if someone is controlling both our hands. For example:

1. If they grab both your wrists tightly, there are some techniques out there where disengaging can work, but when the assailant is significantly bigger and stronger than you they are unfortunately not so easily applied. I have tried all methods and I've found it a much better tactic to relax the wrists being controlled and to use the next available joint as a lever to disengage: in this case, your elbow. This comes as more of a surprise to the grabber, and, combined with a strike, it's very effective and allows you to use minimal effort. If you tense up and start trying to wrestle your wrist out of their hands you will not feel that possibility, and your resistance will lead them to changing their attack.

2. If they grab both your arms above the elbow, you can use exactly the same strategy as above, but this time it's your wrists that are free! So instead of wrestling, use the free parts of your arms (from the elbow down) to disengage.

ATTACK the weak points

It is important to break their thought process and be realistic. If someone has their hands on you and are a threat, but you just try to get them off by using a disengaging technique alone, they can just grab you again. If you create a break in their concentration and shock them by striking at the same time or a fraction before the disengaging technique, the technique itself becomes easier to apply and leaves them distracted for long enough for you to break free.

So attack the targets according to the severity of the situation.

If you are being choked, for example, you have 7–10 seconds before passing out, so you must use that time efficiently: this is a life-or-death situation, a high-level threat, therefore it's appropriate and necessary to attack the weakest targets – the throat and eyes are some of the best options. Remember, disrupting sight and breathing will make the attacker instinctively focus on those areas above all else.

The rule when it comes to a threat is always: STUN/STRIKE, *THEN* DISENGAGE, or ideally DO ALL AT THE SAME TIME. Use the level of force appropriate for the situation.

BREAKING POINTS – grip weaknesses

The wrist and the space between the thumb and the fingers are the weak points of a person's grip, so when attempting to break away we want to apply leverage and pressure to these areas.

We've already looked at how dynamic force can help you disengage from someone's grip (see page 125). This technique below uses the elbow instead to break free by putting pressure on both weak points simultaneously.

The elbow pushes down on the opponent's right wrist, and at the same time we lift our wrist up, breaking the hand free from the loop of their thumb and fingers. You are effectively using your arm like a lever.

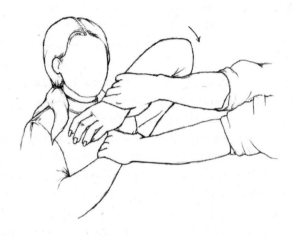

SHORTEST LINE – if they go out, you go in. If they go in, you go out

Just like when we strike, we must make sure we use the shortest line to break out of grabs. Understanding this will allow you to adapt and choose the correct technique.

The laws of physics say that two objects cannot occupy the same space at the same time, so when pitted against a force greater than our own, we need to go where their power is not – so we move our *free* joints in the space that is *not* being occupied.

Another way of expressing this 'shortest line' fighting principle is: 'Where the way is free, flow in.' This has a beautiful philosophical meaning too – it teaches us to notice where we can grow, what we can do and how we can move forward in order to find solutions.

Focusing on the problem we have no power to change will just leave us immobile, wasting valuable time and energy.

For example, if someone is holding both your wrists far apart from each other, you must use your elbow (your free joint) to disengage. But because they are holding your hands wide we have to move the elbow on the inside space between their own arms, using the shortest route. So instead of using the outside route to break, we step in and lift our elbow up as if to try to hit the nose, then push the elbow outwards against one of the grabbing hands (see page 186 for the full technique).

The lesson here is that if you only learn the techniques of self-defence but don't understand the principles, you won't be able to protect yourself against movements with slightly different stances. Someone can grab you with the same hands, in the same place and in the same way but from a slightly wider or closer position, or using a different direction of force, and that can change the technique needed from you. So remembering the principles will help you *find a way*, even if you have not yet tried or seen the technique you need.

This is the difference between a trained mind/programmed body and a programmed mind/trained body. The key is to *train in the techniques* so that our body is programmed with reflexes and *remember the principles* so our mind is able to adapt and find solutions regardless of the situation we may find ourselves in.

GRAB DEFENCES

There are many different techniques you can use to release yourself from a grab, which vary depending on whether the attacker is static or not, and which position they may be holding you in. We'll go into some techniques below using the principles we've learnt earlier in this chapter and throughout the book.

Wrist grabs

Double wrist grab with close hold
If someone grabs both your wrists close to the centre line:

1. Your first action should be to use a strike. Your best options in this scenario are:
   - a whip kick/groin kick (see page 139).
   - a stamp kick to the knee (see page 139).
   - a combination of both – first a whip kick, then a stamp kick. This can be used if the opponent tries to block your groin kick by dipping their knee, leaving you able to attack the knee that has been dipped for you. This is a clear example of taking advantage of what you have and using what they do to your advantage.

2. Immediately after the strike, step in towards your opponent with the same leg without pulling that leg back – just kick and then step. Then use your elbow to disengage: push it up over their arm on the *outside*. When you do this make sure you leave your wrist exactly where it is. Do not pull it back or push it forward, just use your step forward to move your elbow over their grip.

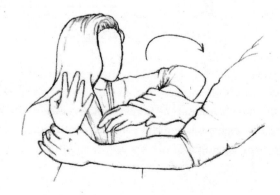

Aim the elbow at the centre of their chest – ideally the sternum; this makes use of your free joint and uses the shortest route. It will also break their grip and leave your opponent with further injury as you've struck a weak target, which gives you more time.

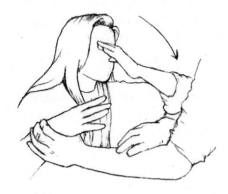

As you push your elbow down, lift your wrist up, using your arm like a lever to free your hand.

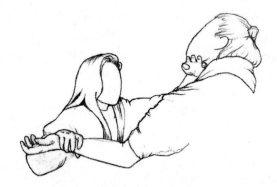

The second your hand is free, use the release to spring to a target, using a chop to the throat with the blade of your hand, for example, and at the same time grab down on the opponent's other wrist.

The static stage is the foundation for practising the technique, but it only becomes an adaptable skill when you practise the technique in motion, learning how to go with your opponent's energy and borrow their force. It becomes a lot easier to apply the technique once you've learnt how to do this, and it puts the opponent at a disadvantage very quickly, because you are moving with their force, rather than responding to it afterwards. Here's how to use different directional forces to your advantage:

Pulling you forward: Use exactly the same technique as the static grab above but just fly in with the elbow much faster. Keep your body and legs under your head to maintain balance, and step to the target catapulting off their force. There may not be time to kick first as the force of the pull may close the distance between you too quickly, so the first strike could be with your knee, or simply use the elbow to simultaneously attack the sternum and disengage.

Pushing you back: As you feel the pressure come towards you, turn sideways and allow their force to continue in the intended direction. At the same time, follow the same technique as the static grab, then follow up with another strike. Because you haven't stopped his force but used it against him, he will fall forward towards the line of your strike. This is what we call double impact – the attacker's force is going in and yours is flying forward. This increases the damage to the target. You'll be striking as soon as they push, so it'll be difficult for them to detect.

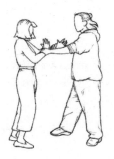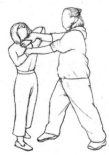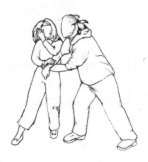

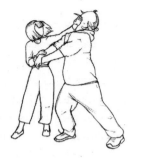 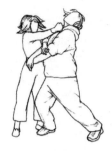

Double wrist grab with wide hold

If they've grabbed both your wrists in a wider position, the way to break their grip will change. The shortest route to break the grip in this scenario is via the centre. That is the free space, so you have to step in.

1. Strike with a free limb (with a whip kick, knee or stamp kick, depending on the distance), then step in with the same leg immediately following the kick.
2. Raise your elbow on the inside line of the grip, the higher the better, and step in at the same time. The main objective here is to get your elbow above their arm so it can be used as a lever to break their grip, but if you are able to strike their nose with your elbow as well that's a useful side-effect. If you used a whip kick beforehand, their head will likely drop and your elbow is more likely to land on a target. Bring your elbow down over their forearm and use it as a lever to break their grip.

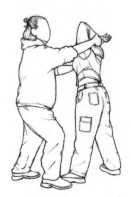

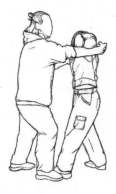 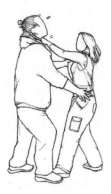

3. Use your free hand to strike another weak target immediately, such as a chop to the throat with the blade of your hand.

Once again, you may need to respond differently here with different directions of force:

Pulling you forward: Because we aim to get close to our opponent in this move anyway, if they pull you in, you just step in with the pull with your elbow raised.

Pushing you back: If they step in towards you, pushing you back, put one leg back as you feel the pressure. Kick or knee with your front leg depending on the distance and then raise your elbow up on the inside of the grab as above (the only difference is that they are closing the distance to you so there is no need to step forward).

Arm grabs

With grabs that are controlling the upper arm we use the lower parts of the arms, which are free to disengage, and the legs.

Double grab on upper arms with close hold

1. Strike the groin with your knee, rotate your hands downwards and step back simultaneously to create space if the person is very close. This gives you more acceleration and force.
2. Once your hands have rotated down and underneath the perpetrator's arms, raise them back up over the outside of their arms and fold them over both of the perpetrator's hands, as if you're about to cross your arms very quickly.
3. Roll your back like a turtle, adding more dynamics to the technique, and draw your hands back towards your chest as you do so – this brings the head of your opponent forward and disengages you from the grab at the same time.
4. Strike a weak target with the blade of your hand as soon as your arms are cleared.

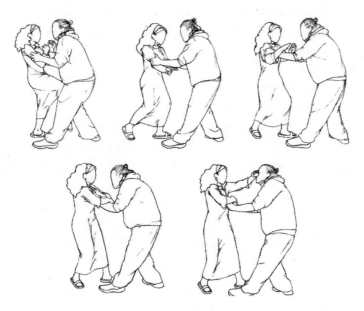

Sexual assault grabs

This might mean a grab to the waist, grabbing you around the arms, pinning both your arms in front of you, or a full-body grab under your arms, with the intention of pulling you in close, either to kiss you or grope you.

Waist grab from the side

1. Give them what they want, just not the way they want it: as they pull you close, lock one of your opponent's legs by hooking your closest foot around their ankle and circling your knee around the outside of their knee (see page 150).

2. With the hand that is closest to them, grab their face from behind, hooking your thumb under their jaw and pushing your fingers into their eyes. Push your knee forwards and tilt their head back at the same time. This creates a lever effect, taking their leg forward and their head back.

3. With your other hand, which should be ready to act at your centre line, strike a weak target. Using the blade of your hand to strike the throat is a good weapon from this position.

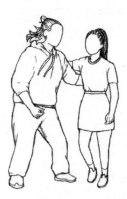 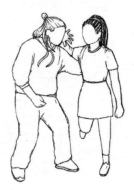

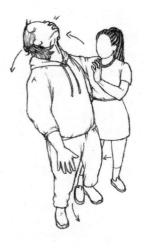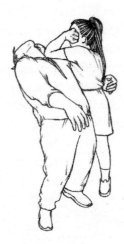

Grab around the arms

1. As above, step in and lock their leg (see page 150) as you feel yourself being pulled in, but this time, because the hand that is closest to them is in front of their grabbing arm, you can use that hand to strike their groin using a reverse palm (see page 141).

2. As soon as you hit the groin, push their knee forward with your knee and as their head drops, using the same hand as before, close your fist and use the back of your elbow in a horizontal backward strike to either their nose or throat (see page 148).

Body grab under the arms from the front

1. As you feel yourself being pulled in, step in with a palm to your attacker's nose, at the same time grabbing their elbow with your other hand and pulling it towards you. This keeps their lower body

from moving back, which makes their head go back further, and also turns them, opening up all the weak targets on the front of their body.

2. Immediately following the palm strike and using the same hand, close your fist, bend your elbow and strike downwards with your elbow (see page 147) on their throat, sternum or solar plexus.

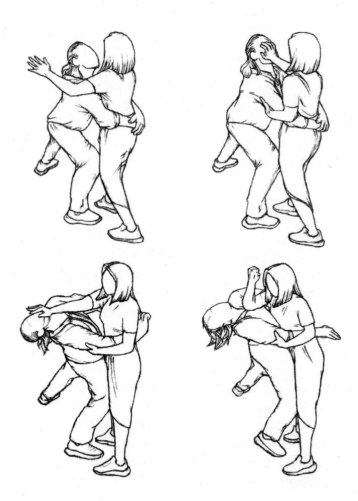

Clothes grabs

Whenever you feel your clothes being pulled and you start to be dragged back, move your legs to keep them centred under your head to keep your balance.

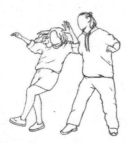

Collar grab from behind

1. As you feel yourself being pulled back, centre your legs under your head.

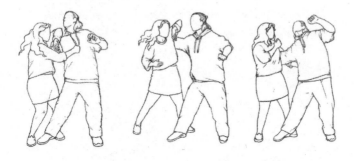

2. Turn your nose to face their nose and at the same time step in and lift one elbow up high enough to cover the side of your face – this is so you can protect your face in case they are intending to strike with the pull. Simultaneously bring your other hand to your centre ready to strike from the shortest line. So three things are happening at once here.

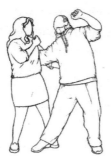 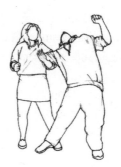

3. As your hand moves forward with your chosen strike to your chosen weak target (an eye strike with thumb, side palm to the throat, front palm to the nose or punch to the throat are all good options here), rotate your raised elbow around the outside of the arm that is grabbing your clothing. Then bring your arm down, squeezing your elbow to your ribs, to trap their grab. This ties up one of their hands for a moment while you initiate the strike.

Hair pulls

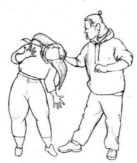

When it comes to hair pulls we have to ensure we keep our legs underneath our head more than ever. If they pull your hair, they can pull your head off the line of your spine very quickly and gain control, putting you in a very compromised position. Again, give them what they want, just not the way they want it:

1. Hold their hand to your head tightly, and push your head against their head, ensuring to push in both directions.

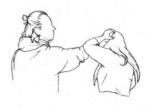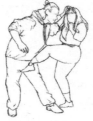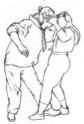

2. Stun them with a strike to cause a break in their concentration and gain control the situation. If you're close you can just use your free hand; if you're far away you can use your legs but follow up with a hand strike.
3. Debilitate their hold. In this case, your opponent's strength is being channelled through their fingers, but you also cannot maintain a strong grab if the muscles you're using to hold on are damaged. So strike with a vertical downward elbow onto their bicep. Ensure your timing is right, as the best and safest time to apply this method is right after your initial strike to their weak targets.

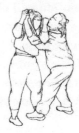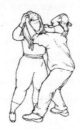

4. Disengage. When someone has their fingers clenched in your hair it is very difficult to pull away. This is why I suggest striking and stunning them, as this will loosen their grip and debilitate them, allowing you to remove yourself from the situation.

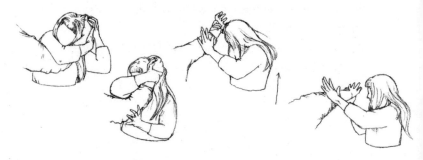

Chokes

This is the most serious type of attack in this category. We need to stop the choke from being effective immediately, by attacking a point that will make the perpetrator automatically change their focus. While removing their hands alone will work with a good technique and if we are just practising in class, a real opponent is likely to grab you again, so you need to *remove the choke* as well as *create injury* in order to escape. Just like with the wrist grabs, we use the shortest-line rule, but as this is a much more serious attack we will use more damaging strikes.

First, here are two vital points to remember:

1. **As soon as a choke is happening you must drop your chin and tense your neck. You will need self-defence techniques to get away, but this first reaction will give you a bit more time.**
2. **Use the fact that they have tied up both of their hands to your advantage and strike weak points. Disturb their vision or airways, as this will**

trigger in the attacker the instinctive response to care for themselves.

- **Nose:** Hit their nose with your palm (see page 141) – if you damage the nose, it messes with their senses, including their sight.
- **Ears:** Cup your hand and hit their ears – this causes excruciating pain and loss of balance.
- **Throat:** Punch them in the throat (see page 142) – if your airways are blocked or injured, nothing is more important! It's the same for your opponent, which makes their throat a prime target. Their instinctive response will be to gasp for air. This gives you time to break free and hopefully get away.
- **Eyes:** Gauge their eyes (see page 146) – if their vision is disturbed little else takes priority.
- **Groin:** Kick or knee their groin (see pages 139 and 145) – this often causes high levels of pain that can bring someone to their knees.

If they slam you into a wall and choke you it's even more serious. If your back is slammed against something solid or you feel yourself pushed backwards, curl forwards, bringing your chin to your chest, and roll your shoulders forward. This will prevent your head from being slammed back, which can knock you unconscious or disorientate you. Keep your legs under your head, as this allows you to feel what's behind you, and you can even use your leg to break the impact.

Narrow choke with their head close

1. If you have the distance, knee their groin. Immediately follow by grabbing their wrist and trapping their arms. An example of this is grabbing their right wrist with your right hand, then raising the elbow on your right arm to be on the outside of their left arm. This will trap both of their hands.
2. Strike down on the sternum with your right elbow as you step in.
3. Follow up with the palm strike to the nose whilst keeping both arms trapped.
4. If you're pushed back in the process, you can use the same method used when a person grabs both your wrists (see page 186) – turn with elbow as leverage and trap with the above technique.

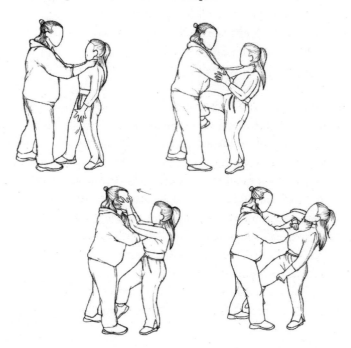

Body grabs

It is important to learn the difference the direction of force makes in body grabs, just as we did with the wrist grabs (see page 186). The grab can look the same but if the attacker is lifting you up or dragging you back, the direction of the force will determine the best response.

In either case, the first and best response to someone trying to pick you up is to ground yourself: make your body limp so it feels like a dead weight. Relax and sink all your energy towards the ground. Then, as soon as you are able to, use a strike aimed at weak targets.

The body grab from behind is most commonly used to lift and carry someone to a secondary location rather than just stand still and hold them. So if you can ground your weight first and quickly implement a reverse palm (see page 141), this can prevent the lift altogether with the right timing. If you don't manage that, do the following if they lift you, or if they put you back down, even if only for a moment.

Lifting abduction from behind

1. As soon as you feel anyone's arms around you, sink to the floor and adopt a base stance by grounding your weight and widening your legs as if you want to sit on the ground. This makes you a lot heavier and more difficult to lift, so they may put you back down for a moment or struggle more, all of which gives you time and opportunity to strike back, then disengage.
2. If you do not have time or space to strike, use your feet as anchors by hooking them around the base of the attacker's legs or knees. Even if it's just one, this is still effective. You can anchor your foot on the outside or inside of their leg; the best hooking point is their knees, as they are usually bent when trying to gain force to lift, and the best time to do this is while

they are static, trying to lift you. Then, as you are a
bit more elevated, you can use your free leg to
heel-kick their groin. This is a great tactic as most
who want to abduct need to do so in a hurry, so
making the process long, exhausting and difficult can
result in them aborting the abduction. Hooking their
legs can prevent them moving you to a secondary
location and can result in them tripping, or just
having to put you down again and try again, which
gives you an opportunity to strike.

3. When you do have space and time, use strikes with
the weapons you have available. If your hands are
free because they lifted you under your arms, and
their head is within range, use the backs of your
elbows to strike their head. Alternatively, if they are
very tall and their head is far away, use cupped palms
to smack their ears from behind. If they grab over
your arms, you can use a reverse palm to their groin
(see page 141).

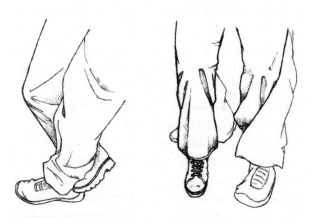

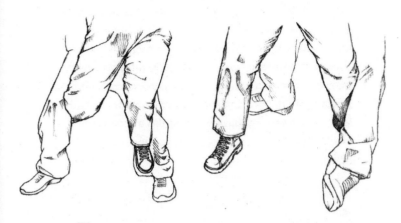

Static body grab under the arms from behind

1. When your feet are in contact with the floor – if the attack is static (i.e. they are holding you but not pulling or lifting you) or if the person trying to lift you puts you back down for a moment – ground your weight and adopt the wide base stance, and as you do this grab their arm that is crossed over your body by the wrist and pull it to one side (if you grab their right wrist with your left hand, pull it to your left, and vice versa) as this sets you up for the next move.

2. Move your hips to one side, in this case your left, step out a little (if moving your hips to the left, step out with your left leg) and in the space that has opened up swing your right hand back in a reverse palm to the groin (see page 141).

3. Immediately following this strike, step behind their leg (if you moved your hips to the left then step behind their left leg using your right leg as the space is already there. Use a leg lock (see page 150) and at the same time aim a right horizontal backward elbow

(see page 148) at their head, which is now in range because we have moved to a better position and the groin shot will encourage an instinctive reaction in them to bend their lower body back and their head forward. The mechanics of striking their head and pushing their knee at the same time makes their grab very unstable and gives you the opportunity to escape.

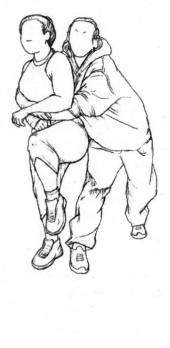

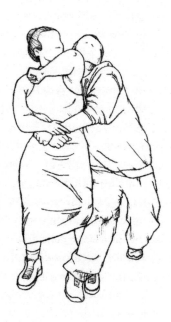

11.

GROUND DEFENCE BASICS
(IMMINENT DANGER: PART 4)

Ground defence is a very large topic – there are entire systems based upon it – however, it is important to grasp the basics, so I have laid out some tactics and simple techniques that can be useful on the ground.

Let's first look at the different levels of ground defence and the scenarios they represent regarding you and your attacker:

Level 1: You are both standing, and they are trying to get you to the ground.

Level 2: You are on the ground and they are standing, and you need to prevent their attack from a close distance with your first lines of ground defence: your front and rear legs.

Level 3: You are both on the ground, and they are past your first lines of ground defence. You are now relying on your knees.

Level 4: They have broken through your lines of ground defence (both of your legs and your knees).

The areas we will cover in this chapter are:
- Prevention when standing.
- How to prevent the attacker from getting close to you, around you or through your legs when you are on the ground and the attacker is standing.
- How to stop the attacker getting close to your side or between your legs when they are also on the ground.
- What to do if the attacker manages to get between your legs.

....

There are many ways you can use being on the ground to your advantage, although it is a position we want to avoid getting into if possible. You are less mobile on the floor, and you have to get back up before you can get away, which could be particularly difficult if you do fall, as this can cause injury. So first we have to learn ways to make it difficult for someone to get you on the ground to begin with.

LEVEL 1: THEY ARE TRYING TO GET YOU DOWN

When a person is pulled, pushed or dragged to the ground it means they have either lost balance, tripped over something or their head has been taken off the line of the spine by use of force, such as being pushed back, having their hair pulled, or being dragged or struck down.

If someone pulls your clothes or hair to drag you down, you can pin the hands they're using in place and keep your legs under your head.

In Chapter 10: Controlling Attackers we looked at how to deal with clothes grabs and hair pulls, which may be intended to drag you down, and we saw how essential it was to keep your head in line with your spine and your legs so as not to lose your balance. This will buy you time and make it a lot harder for them to pull you to the ground. Let's imagine three scenarios to illustrate how useful this is:

1. You are pushed from behind
As you feel your upper-body weight go forward, step with the push – almost like a big lunge – keeping your knee under your head. If the push is really big, you can do as many steps as needed to catch up with your head, but once you can do the lunge-like step this can restabilise you. As soon as you have balance on that leg you can use it to either spring further forward before turning to see where your opponent is or run to safety. When you do turn, make sure your hands are at your centre in preparation. If your attacker is right behind you, lift your elbow as you turn as in the clothes grab technique and shoot a strike from the centre line with your other hand.

2. You are in a headlock
There are different techniques for managing a headlock at every level, from when you are first standing to when you're almost horizontally bent over, which are beyond the scope of this book to cover, but initially the way to prevent it from moving your head from the 12 o'clock to 1 o'clock position is to walk with it, keeping your legs under your head and standing up straight. This is the best position from which to administer the numerous disengagement techniques available.

3. You are shoved back from the front
Step back with the force (again, this may mean your legs change position a few times). Once your head is aligned with your legs, ground your weight on your back leg and at the same time lift your hands to the centre in a semi-circular motion on the inside of their push in two beggar's palms (see page 102), so that they hover over their elbows, then turn your hands over, grab their elbows and pull. You can then aim a kick at their groin (see page 139), or stamp kick their front leg (see page 139), followed by a palm strike (see page 141), or even a chain of palm strikes, to their nose.

HOW TO FALL SAFELY

If you feel you're losing your balance and there is no contact with the attacker at this point, you need to protect yourself from the ground so as to suffer as few injuries as possible.

Try to push your head forward and tuck your chin to your chest with your mouth closed. If your feet are still on the ground, bend your knees as if to sit or place one foot back and bend that knee. As you go down try to create a turtle-shell shape with your back and cross your hands over your chest or hold them at the centre of your body in the guard position, so you do not have the urge to slam them down to break your fall.

As you feel yourself rolling back on the ground, you can place your palms at the sides of your body to help break the fall, but only do this at the last second. This is a Brazilian jiu-jitsu way of breaking a fall, which I found really helpful.

LEVEL 2: YOU ARE ON THE GROUND, THEY ARE STANDING

If you are on the floor and have good enough distance, get up as soon as you can while keeping at least one hand forward, in case of incoming blows. If there is not enough distance and the attacker is steadily approaching, you need to get into a strong position and create lines of defence from the ground.

Adopt the ground guard position

There are two options when it comes to creating a guard position from the ground, depending on how close your attacker is:

Option 1: Open-leg guard
This is a very strong position that uses both your legs to control the

legs of your opponent, and is best used if the person is very close. Keep your legs on your attacker's hips and, once they are close enough for you to reach, hook your hands on the outside of their ankles and pull them towards you while pushing your heels against their hips. This is a very effective way to drop someone. As soon as they are down, use your heel to kick their groin, then get up quickly.

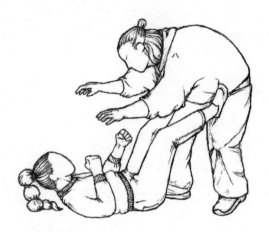

Option 2: Two lines of defence guard

This option is best when you have a little more distance from your attacker and follows the same strategy as when we are standing, setting up double guard positions with both your hands and your legs. Keep your chin tucked in and your hands in the guard position on your centre line. Keep one leg bent with your foot firmly on ground and the other up, with knee bent, facing your opponent, ready to fire a kick if they come within range. Turn the raised foot slightly so your toes are facing outwards, because you will likely be kicking your attacker's knees and are more likely not to slide off target if your foot is almost horizontal. Here, the nose-to-nose theory is again vital: keep your nose, hands and feet all in one line facing your opponent.

This option will now give five lines of defence in total:

- Front leg
- Rear leg
- Knee line
- Front hand
- Rear hand

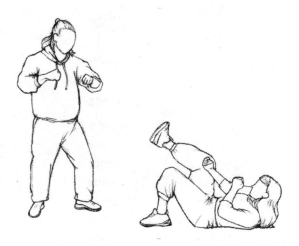

Be aware of your magnetic distance

This theory applies when you are on the ground and your legs are facing your opponent. As soon as they come within your magnetic distance, which is your kicking range, you have to attack their weak targets. In this case we are looking to inflict pain to the knees, groin and ankles. If they bend their head down this will also be in range as another target.

Magnetic distance stems from the legend of the crane, just like the nose-to-nose method (see page 123). Imagine your striking foot is the crane's beak: ensure this is always pointing towards your opponent if you're on the ground.

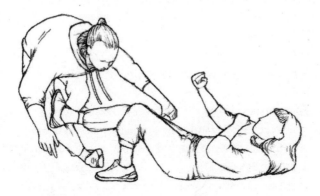

Stay nose to nose

If your attacker tries to get to the side of you by changing direction, pivot on the ground keeping your nose on their nose, just as you would when standing. The only difference here is that your guard is your legs, too, so keep them at your centre, in line with their centre, as you move. Every time they try to get around you, adjust to keep yourself in front of them. If they step in, this is when you kick using your magnetic distance as discussed above.

Use 'bamboo legs'

For ground defence work, do not keep your legs too stiff or too floppy – they need to be kept both strong and flexible like springs! Keep your knees bent as this will allow you to strike from where you are, rather than having to pull back. Just like with bamboo, any push and pull when using this technique will allow your legs to spring back.

First line of defence: Front leg

Your legs are your main lines of defence when you're on the ground. Use your front leg to rotate and kick (making sure your foot is horizontal when kicking narrow leg targets), aiming for knees and ankles, and, if needed, swap your front and rear legs to fire more kicks if one is compromised.

If they grab your front ankle and try to drag you

1. As soon as you feel the grab on your front leg, place your rear foot horizontally on their closest ankle, right at the base, and push it away while pulling your front leg towards you. This works like a finger trap; the more they pull, the more stuck they are. As soon as you feel the initial jolt stopping their pull, jump the rear foot that's on their ankle up to their knee and stamp kick it (see page 139).

2. At this point you have two options to disengage:

- If the grab is with both hands and their arms are wide, hook the heel of your kicking foot over their closest arm and pull it down to clear that hand, and at the same time pull your front leg back, freeing it from their other hand. As soon as one leg is clear, you can aim a kick to a weak target, such as their head if it's in range.

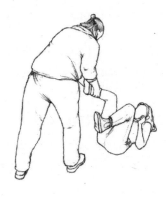

- If they grab with one hand or both hands very close together, after the kick to the knee place that foot on the floor to gain stability and at the same time circle the front foot that is being grabbed. Use your toes to circle over their wrists and then push your foot down on the outside. This places pressure on their wrists – the weakest part of their grab – and releases your foot.

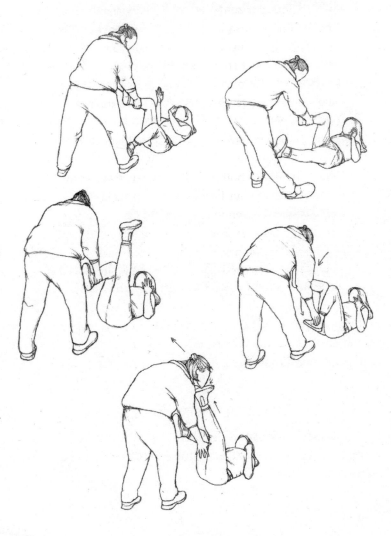

Second line of defence: Rear leg

If the attacker moves quickly to get past your front leg and tries to get round the side of you, you can pivot and switch legs to keep up with them. This will make it more difficult for them to get around you.

If the attacker gets past your front leg

1. If they slap or push your raised front leg to the side in an attempt to get between your legs, immediately change legs.
2. When you bring your rear leg forward fire a kick at their knees or ankles, unless their face or chest is in range, in which case you can target those instead.
3. If they are stepping to the inside of your left leg, their weight will likely be placed on their left leg to move in that direction, so pivot in line with them and stamp that left knee with your right leg. Keep your nose in line with theirs and use your magnetic distance to strike when they're in range.

LEVEL 3: YOU ARE BOTH ON THE GROUND, PAST YOUR FIRST LINES OF DEFENCE

In this situation you are less mobile and in a compromised position on the ground, so any moves beyond the example below would require advanced training.

Third line of defence: Knees

Your attacker is now close enough to grab your body. Below is an example of how to prevent them getting any closer to you, using your knees as your prime weapon:

If they try to get between your legs

1. Use your hands to deflect theirs, then hold one knee at a 90-degree angle and push it into their ribs. Push from your back towards your opponent, maintaining a barrier between you.
2. Use what they're doing to your advantage. If they're focusing on opening your legs and keep grabbing them, use your strikes and everyday objects (see page 130) to create time and space, and cause injury. Always strike their weak targets as and when you can.
3. Keep your legs moving so it's difficult for the opponent to control them.

LEVEL 4: THEY ARE INSIDE YOUR LINES OF GROUND DEFENCE

If you are both on the ground and your attacker has broken through all your lines of defence, this is a very uncomfortable and frightening position to be in, but you do still have options. Your body and possibly your hands are your weapons here, as in the example below. Bear in mind, however, that Level 4 defence is an advanced area so any further advice would require professional in-person training.

Fourth line of defence: Body/hands

If the attacker is already between your legs, you can use the closed guard position to turn the situation to your advantage.

If they get between your legs

1. Wrap your legs around their waist and squeeze, crossing your ankles and using your hips to push them back. This gives you control of their core, as your hips are very strong.
2. If your hands are free keep them in the guard position in case of oncoming blows and use the strategies you have learned – the bridging arm technique, for example, would work well here (see page 166) – to create time and space to get away.
3. If the attacker is trying to exhaust you by laying their torso on yours, place both palms on their collar bones, push your back into the ground and lock your arms, creating a wedge between you and them. This will give you some space to push your hips to one side; if you move your hips to the left, place your right foot on the centre of their hips and push yourself back off their weight. Stamp kick a weak target, such as their face with your free leg, which will give you the time and space to get off the ground safely and find safety.

....

Fighting principles are adaptable even on the ground, and for me this is a vital part of self-defence. I was six years into my career when I learned ground fighting for the first time; I felt it was the missing link to a lot of what I had already learned, and I am still fascinated by the topic. Not all self-defence clubs teach it, but there are specialist clubs you can sign up to that cover the topic extensively. For more information on ground defence and where best to learn it please see Chapter 12: Your Training and Resources.

12.

YOUR TRAINING

When you think about it, it is counterproductive to learn how to defend yourself from others if you are not aware of or willing to address the things you may be doing that are harming yourself.

We naturally support, nurture and encourage our loved ones to look after themselves, but many of us find it hard to treat ourselves with the same love and respect. Self-love is definitely part of self-defence; traditionally it's just been explained differently – as training your mind, body and spirit.

Practising martial arts is so beneficial and empowering when taught holistically, as a whole and under healthy guidance, which is why for many it can be used as a way of life, not just as a means to survive. If you are healthier, it impacts on the regulation of your emotions. If you are physically fit you are stronger, quicker and more agile. And if you are spiritually aligned with your authentic self then you will *trust* yourself to find solutions in difficult situations. So in your training, try to cover all the areas of development: mental, physical and spiritual.

MENTAL DEVELOPMENT

Martial arts, self-defence and many other activities and forms of exercise have the capacity to improve our mental health, reduce depression and enhance our mood by releasing some or all of the four happy hormones – the chemicals in the brain that create a feeling of wellbeing. Below is a summary of what those hormones do and how you can help boost their production:

Dopamine is known as the reward hormone. It can be increased by setting and achieving small and regular goals. It improves memory, motivation, attention, focus and the regulation of body movements. Practising martial arts in a grading system that encourages you to test and develop your abilities, signing up to a short course on a topic you are interested in, doing weekly yoga classes, joining a fitness challenge or learning a new language will all boost this hormone and the benefits that come along with it.

Oxytocin is more commonly known as the love hormone but it's essentially a bonding chemical. It can be released or increased through intimacy but also through socialising. Being part of a new group doing some recreational activities will expose you to people with similar interests, but also just talking, going for a walk or stroking a dog can encourage this happy hormone.

Serotonin is known for regulating sleep and appetite. It promotes positive feelings and is linked to our gut. This is why when we feel stressed or anxious we can experience stomach issues. Exercise is one of the ways to boost it, and it can also be increased from being out in the sun.

Endorphins regulate the fight-or-flight instinct and are your body's way of providing natural pain relief when needed. Physical exercise and meditative practices like chi kung increase the production of endorphins, as do activities that make you laugh and even eating chocolate.

In many ways these kinds of activities can enhance our ability to function in our daily lives and navigate through the difficult times. And it works like a cycle – when we feel better in our minds we are more likely to make healthier decisions for our bodies and our lifestyle. Whether it's through therapy, meditation, learning to set healthy boundaries, self-care, exercise or nurturing friendships and relationships, looking after your mental health will help your martial arts training to develop, improving your grasp of the strategies and tactics and fighting principles that underpin the practice. And in turn your martial arts training will help you look after your mental health, building a sense of resilience, empowerment, self-belief and – one of the most important tools to success – discipline. Discipline helps us do the things we know are good for us even if we do not feel motivated. It helps us be consistent, and if you are consistent at anything you are more likely to succeed.

PHYSICAL DEVELOPMENT

First, before embarking on any kind of new exercise training, you should understand your physical limitations, which could be determined by illnesses, injuries or disabilities. This will allow you to adapt what you learn to your own circumstances and capabilities. Yet regardless of your physical fitness, there are always certain things you can do to give yourself a helping hand and ensure you are as fit and healthy as you can possibly be.

Health

Health includes nutrition and looking after your body, so always take care to eat well, sleep well and drink plenty of water. It's not for me to tell you what to do with your life or question your life choices, but I do encourage you to consider your health as a priority. If you want to learn how to defend yourself it means you want to feel and be safe, which is a way of being kind to yourself. Abstaining from things that can severely harm your health is an excellent way to start, so here are some examples of substances that adversely affect our health and our ability to defend ourselves:

- **Alcohol** directly affects the nervous system. I have felt this myself when I have been out for cocktails with friends. The next day I can instantly feel that my speed and reflexes are a little slower. I now know not to drink when I am training the next day or when I am in a period of training constantly. Many times I've gone teetotal for long periods, even years, though that isn't always necessary. Moderation is advisable, and it's important to know how it can affect you.
- **Smoking** damages your lungs – we all know that. The dangers of smoking can be seen everywhere now. Bad lung health will directly impact on your ability to perform, as you need energy and oxygen to move. If you are a smoker or ex-smoker, yoga and chi kung are great ways to help your lungs heal, as they improve the immune system and the breathing exercises help increase lung capacity. I used to smoke, and when I started training I would often get lightheaded and tire out easily. Chi kung helped me get more oxygen into my lungs and regulate my breathing. I also have mild asthma, but I have only had to use my pump once in 16 years since I started practising chi kung.

Fitness

Look after your body and invest in physical fitness. This could mean any number of activities, from walking, running, swimming or joining a gym to taking up yoga or dance. Anything that encourages movement that works with your lifestyle and physical abilities will work towards improving your general fitness, and in turn it will increase your energy and stamina and boost your mood.

Joining a self-defence class or martial arts club can of course be part of this. When choosing a club to join, make sure you agree with their ethos and their approach; do your research and *check reviews*. Look out for clubs that are inclusive and have some female instructors. I would avoid clubs with a misogynistic vibe, particularly if you are a survivor, as that environment can feel quite triggering. Look for reviews by women.

You can ask for a trial lesson to get a feel of the place. Read what their club rules are and keep in mind that you can always ask to just watch the first lesson. Styles that rely on physics, kinetic force and geometry will allow you to develop skills that aren't dependent on force, size or ability. Wing Tsun is one of those styles, which is why I've focused so much of my training on it, but you can research other systems that also use those principles.

For ground defence work Brazilian jiu-jitsu is a fantastic route! As a useful addition to your defence and strike techniques, consider working on other forms physical training, such as shadow boxing, pad work drills, sparring and reflex training. These will all help improve your speed, agility, strength and reactions.

SPIRITUAL DEVELOPMENT

As we discussed earlier in the book, effective self-defence is as much about mindset as it is about physical technique, so working on your spiritual development should be a key element in your training.

Internal work

Practise connecting with yourself through introspection, mindfulness and journaling. These are all healthy ways to develop and understand yourself internally. Meditative practices such as yoga and chi kung can also promote clarity of thought and mental balance. Look back at Chapter 2: Mental Discernment and Self-belief for more on how to build your sense of self, regulate your internal dialogue, develop a powerful mindset and connect with your fighting spirit.

....

Remember, when working through your training, try to cover all the pillars of development for a fully holistic approach to get the best out of your experience:

Mental Development: Mental Health, Awareness, Discernment, Clarity, Setting Boundaries, Meditation, Yoga, Physical Activity, Strategies and Tactics, Fighting Principles

Physical Development: Exercise, Sleep, Nutrition, Water, Training Strikes and Techniques, Pad Work Drills, Shadow Boxing, Reflex Training, Sparring

Spiritual Development: Introspection, Internal Dialogue, Mindfulness, Journaling, Mindset, Self-belief, Self-awareness, the Art of Acceptance, Meditation, Yoga, Chi Kung

CONCLUSION

Every new skill starts with 'a little idea' and the courage to take the first step.

I hope you have found value in this book as that first step. For some, this may be something you want to reflect back on from time to time, and for others it may be an introduction to something new.

This is the first book I have written, and although I enjoy writing, I have never taught self-defence through a book before, so this was a new and interesting journey for me. I cannot see any of your faces or know you like I normally would if you were to attend one of my classes, but I do hope that my method, knowledge and heart as a teacher has come through these pages in a way that has been helpful.

At first, I wanted to show everything, to make sure that every corner and every turn possible was covered, but any good teacher knows that too much information can be as bad as none at all, so finding this balance was important. To do that, I tried to stay centred and focused on the purpose, and I used the very principles I've written about to help me navigate through this uncharted territory. It has been pretty affirming to learn how useful those principles are in all kinds of challenges.

The most important thing to me is that you can now see that there is indeed a very practical way in which we can defend ourselves regardless of our size, age or gender. That we can protect ourselves if needed, physically, mentally and spiritually.

I hope you can also now see that there is a difference between being aware and being on high alert, and that we can be aware in a healthy way that feels good and helpful. That fear is not something we need to overcome or push down, but something we can appropriate. And that being *told* by those in power that we need to do this or that in order to solve the issues surrounding our safety is very different to seeking out advice or tools on how to learn a new skill. One is your prerogative, the other is victim blaming. The interest in learning self-defence should never cancel out the understanding that we shouldn't have to learn it. Remember that self-defence gives you a chance to protect yourself if needed and *if all else fails*. That doesn't mean it's okay for us to continue to be failed by society. We all deserve safety.

So this book is for you and not a means to tackle systemic social issues. My aim was to give you your own personal guide, a way for you to learn and find useful information, and to show that you can be empowered by that.

Knowing how to protect yourself and how to develop awareness, a strong mentality, confidence in setting boundaries and the ability to spot red flags and respond with composure under pressure are all empowering tools that are useful in all areas of life. But you should only seek to learn them if you feel they are *for you*, and that they will make *you* feel good.

I also hope my intention to inspire readers to see the beauty in martial arts has been successful. I wanted to show that it's so much more than self-defence – that it can be a way of life and not just for survival.

There are many ways to reach a destination, but this way has been most helpful and empowering to me. I wish I'd had some of this knowledge earlier, but that is why I am sharing it here with you now. It has truly been an honour to write this book and share these teachings with you.

AFFIRMATIONS

FIGHTING LIKE A GIRL IS ...

... saying that 'like a girl' is no longer an insult, but a reflection of strength, resilience and power.

... your prerogative, something you do because you want to and can do, and not because you believe you should.

... showing up for yourself as your authentic self.

... having a 'last arrow' should you need one.

... not changing your behaviour so that perpetrators do not have to.

... letting go of what no longer serves us.

... an alternative path to empowerment.

... saying it's okay to feel fear, but we will no longer be running on it.

... making the most of what you have and realising all that you can be.

... for self-empowerment and self-defence, never for revenge.

... utilising all that is accessible and natural to us.

... not imitating another but accessing the best version of yourself.

... being aware, present and centred, without running on high alert.

... intelligence over brute force.

... knowing that fear and aggression are appropriate, so long as we are not running on them.

... knowing that violence is fighting with the absence of justice, but self-defence is fighting with the presence of it.

....

Fighting like a girl has no place for misogyny or any forms of bias.

Fighting like a girl understands the difference between victim blaming and being prepared.

RESOURCES

Video recordings of techniques mentioned in this book and more have been uploaded to http://www.fightlikeagirluk.org/tutorials. These are free for all readers to access using password equanimity.

WHERE TO FIND ME

- Fight Like a Girl UK: www.fightlikeagirluk.org
- Phoenix Eye Wing Tsun Association: www.phoenixeyewingtsunlondon.co.uk
- www.allianceforwingtsun.com

DOMESTIC VIOLENCE SERVICES

- Southwark Bede House: www.bedehouse.org.uk
- Women's Aid: www.womensaid.org.uk
- Refuge: www.refuge.org.uk

SUPPORT AGAINST STALKER SERVICES

- National Stalking Helpline: 0808 802 0300
- Protection Against Stalking: www.protectionagainststalking.org
- UK Revenge Porn Helpline: 0345 6000 459 https://revengepornhelpline.org.uk/

PERSONAL SAFETY

- How to make a silent 999 call:
  www.met.police.uk/contact/how-to-make-a-silent-999-call/
- How to use Emergency SOS on your iPhone:
  https://support.apple.com/en-gb/HT208076
- What3words app – a way to identify your precise location
  using a unique combination of three words:
  https://what3words.com

SELF-DEFENCE CLUBS

- Phoenix Eye Wing Tsun Association:
  www.phoenixeyewingtsunlondon.co.uk
- EBMAS (UK and Ireland)
- Carpe Diem BBJ London – Brazilian Jiu Jitsu academy,
  based on ground work: www.carpediembjj.co.uk/
- Triccs Academy – teaches Brazilian jiu-jitsu, based on
  ground work: www.dulwichbjj.com
- Dr Jon Xue – FLAG team member, instructor and ally,
  stunt man, actor, martial artist and metaphysician:
  www.xue-zhang.com
- Nick Chand – hosts FLAG workshops in Wolverhampton:
  info@aikidobodoalliance.org
- IMAS Wing Chun (Vik Hothi) – www.imas-uk.com
- Sifu Terry (Harrogate) – www.wtmartialartsharrogate.co.uk
- Sifu Mark Carson – Bangor Ireland:
  www.schoolofeverything.com/teacher/markcarson

MENTAL HEALTH SUPPORT

- NHS mental health services: www.nhs.uk/mental

YOGA

- Elumi Yoga: www.elumiyoga.co.uk
- Sadhana Yoga & Wellbeing: https://sadhana-wellbeing.com/

RECOMMENDED BOOKS

This book is about self-defence, but if you are interested in learning about the many very real issues that impact on society there are some great books out there written by amazing and well-informed authors who are really flying the flag for progressiveness and equality. These are some of the books that I always go back to, that have really helped and inspired me, and given me some amazing life tools.

- *Be Water, My Friend: The True Teachings of Bruce Lee* by Shannon Lee (Rider, 2020)
- *Dao De Jing: The Book of the Way* by Lao Tzu (University of California Press, 2002)
- *Fix the System, Not the Women* by Laura Bates (Simon & Schuster, 2022)
- *Girl Up* by Laura Bates (Simon & Schuster, 2016)
- *Men Who Hate Women: The Extremism Nobody Is Talking About* by Laura Bates (Simon & Schuster, 2021)
- *Misogynoir Transformed: Black Women's Digital Resistance* by Moya Bailey (New York University, 2021)
- *Nei Kung: The Secret Teachings of the Warrior Sages* by Kosta Danaos (Inner Traditions, 2002)

- *The Art of Peace* by Morihei Ueshiba (Shambhala Publications Inc., 2007)
- *The Art of War* by Sun Tzu (Pax Librorum, 2009)
- *The Journeys of Socrates* by Dan Millman (HarperOne, 2006)
- *The Subtle Art of Not Giving a F**k: A Counterintuitive Approach to Living a Good Life* by Mark Manson (Harper, 2016)
- *This Book Is Anti-racist: 20 Lessons on How to Wake Up, Take Action and Do the Work* by Tiffany Jewell and Aurelia Durand (Frances Lincoln, 2020)
- *This Book Is Feminist: An Intersectional Primer for Next-Gen Changemakers* by Jamia Wilson and Aurelia Durand (Frances Lincoln, 2021)
- *Way of the Peaceful Warrior: A Book That Changes Lives* by Dan Millman (Sounds True, 2017)

ACKNOWLEDGEMENTS

Thank you to all the women who inspired me to set up FLAG, and all who have supported the women's self-defence workshops and courses, and given their expert advice and feedback: Elizabeth Chung (FLAG women's self-defence instructor); Ann Clark (FLAG women's self-defence instructor); Si-Mo Sapphyre Haynes; Lorena Mondonico; Bede House women's domestic violence services – Nicole, Ahlam, Habiba; Sifu József Bányász (leader of Zenit Wing Tsun, Hungary); Tamás Barta (leader of Vamillion Wing Tsun, Hungary); Kerry Howard, for providing expert feedback on Chapters 2 and 4; Eliza Ioannou of Elumi Yoga for content in Chapter 4; Dr Jon Xue (FLAG team member) for providing expert advice, guidance and feedback on Chapter 3; Sifu Emin Boztepe (leader of EBMAS); Mark Stas (leader of Wing Flow system); Simon Alebiosu (business support and personal trainer at Beyond Balance Inc.); Si-Hing Joseph Parker (FLAG and Phoenix Eye instructor); Doug Southall (photographer at Pepper Pictures); my agent Philippa Sitters – thank you for asking me to write this book; Sifu Vik Hothi (hosts FLAG workshops in Slough); Nick Chand (hosts FLAG workshops in Wolverhampton); Becky (illustrator); Anna and Julia (editors at HarperCollins); Si-Je Asha Tullet (photography); Si-Hing Chris Tullet (photography); Si-Hing Michael McGinley (photography); Roxanne and Dominic Haslam – for feedback, advice and support; Arriel Smith (photography).

Thank you for being supportive: Helen O'Sullivan – I dedicate this book to you, and I will love you always; Patrick O'Sullivan – for all that you do and have done; Jayden O'Sullivan – I love you, son; Ryan O'Sullivan – for introducing me to martial arts; Sensei George Andrews of Okinawan Traditional Goju Ryu Karate-do Association – my first ever martial arts teacher; Sifu Arthur Haynes (Phoenix

Eye teacher); Sifu Bill Cooper (Phoenix Eye teacher); Sifu Mark Stas; Sifu Carson Lau; Lois Jacobs; Nick Knowles for your constant support – thanks for always believing in me; and all my students, my friends and my family.

NOTES

1   World Health Organization, on behalf of the United Nations Inter-Agency Working Group on Violence Against Women Estimation and Data (2021).

2   Chaka L. Bachmann and Becca Gooch, 'LGBT in Britain: Hate Crime and Discrimination', YouGov/Stonewall report (2017): https://www.stonewall.org.uk/system/files/lgbt_in_britain_hate_crime.pdf

3   Joan Didion, 'On Keeping a Notebook', *Slouching Towards Bethlehem* (Farrar, Straus and Giroux, 1968).

4   A. J. Adams, 'Seeing Is Believing: The Power of Visualization', *Psychology Today*, 3 December 2009: https://www.psychologytoday.com/gb/blog/flourish/200912/seeing-is-believing-the-power-visualization

5   Suzanne Rowan Kelleher, 'Why You Should Start Screening for Hidden Spy Cameras When You Travel', *Forbes*, 27 January 2020: https://www.forbes.com/sites/suzannerowankelleher/2020/01/27/why-you-should-start-screening-for-hidden-spy-cameras-when-you-travel/amp/

6   Jill Yaworski, 'The Sound That Will Make You 7 Percent Stronger', *Men's Health* (12 November 2012): https://www.menshealth.com/fitness/a19533055/the-sound-that-will-make-you-7-percent-stronger/

7   Chun-Yi Lin et al., 'Acute Physiological Effects if Qigong Exercise in Older Practitioners', *Evidence-based Complementary and Alternative Medicine* (April 2018): doi: 10.1155/2018/4960978

8   Jill E. Bormann et al., 'Individual Treatment of Posttraumatic Stress Disorder Using Mantram Repetition: A Randomized Clinical Trial', *American Journal of Psychiatry*, 175: 10 (June 2018), 979–88: https://doi.org/10.1176/appi.ajp.2018.17060611; Gemma Perry et al., 'Chanting Meditation Improves Mood and Social Cohesion', Proceedings of the 14th International Conference on Music Perception and Cognition

(July 2016): https://www.researchgate.net/publication/319851087_
Chanting_Meditation_Improves_Mood_and_Social_Cohesion

9   Femicide Census 2020: https://www.femicidecensus.org/wp-content/
uploads/2022/02/010998-2020-Femicide-Report_V2.pdf; https://www.
endviolenceagainstwomen.org.uk/femicide-census-reveals-half-of-uk-
women-killed-by-men-die-at-hands-of-partner-or-ex/

10 Suzy Lamplugh Trust, 'What Is Stalking?': https://www.suzylamplugh.
org/what-is-stalking

11 Lorraine Sheridan et al., 'The Course and Nature of Stalking: A Victim
Perspective', *Howard Journal of Crime and Justice*, 40: 3 (August 2001),
215–34: DOI:10.1111/1468-2311.00204

12 National Stalking Helpline, 2011.

13 This was established by the following case in 1983: (*R v Williams (G)
78 Cr App R 276*), (*R. v Oatbridge, 94 Cr App R 367*).

14 Criminal Law Act 1967. If you do not live in the UK, you can check
the current laws regarding pre-emptive strike and self-defence that
apply to where you live.

15 WomensMedia, 'What the Vagus Nerve Is and How to Stimulate It for
Better Mental Health', *Forbes* (15 April 2021): https://www.forbes.com/
sites/womensmedia/2021/04/15/what-the-vagus-nerve-is-and-how-to-
stimulate-it-for-better-mental-health/?sh=779f4dc56250

16 Jill Yaworski, 'The Sound That Will Make You 7 Percent Stronger',
Men's Health (12 November 2012): https://www.menshealth.com/
fitness/a19533055/the-sound-that-will-make-you-7-percent-stronger/

ABOUT THE AUTHOR

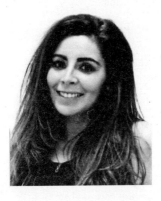

Della O'Sullivan is a women's self-defence expert, weapons expert and leading UK martial artist. She studies more than one style of martial arts but has obtained the level of 'master' in Wing Tsun kung fu, and is also currently working towards a degree in criminology and psychology. Della has become an advocate for female empowerment after revealing her inspirational journey through martial arts as a survivor of violence. She supports domestic violence charities, and in 2016 she launched her Fight Like a Girl campaign in support of the Bede House charity, where workshops were set up across London at women-only centres to to assist other survivors and encourage more women to see the benefits of martial arts and self-defence. She has taught hundreds of women since launching the campaign.

Della started teaching martial arts in 2007 after training for the equivalent average hours of four years in one. She opened her first school in Dulwich, South London, where she continues to teach, and has led countless public demonstrations both in the UK and abroad. In 2011, she performed on stage to a packed audience at the Shaolin Temple in Dengfeng, China, alongside the legendary Shaolin monks. She has also appeared in several newspaper articles and was featured in London's *Evening Standard*, on the BBC's *The*

One Show, Radio 4 and the ITV evening news. She has featured in a BBC documentary about positive female role models and was the subject of a special feature in *Martial Arts Illustrated* and *Wing Chun Illustrated*. As well as offering self-defence classes for various councils and being a guest teacher for other martial art schools, charitable organisations and universities, she also teaches regular martial arts classes to men, women and children within her own Phoenix Eye Wing Tsun Association.

'In an ideal world a woman should feel okay walking into any martial arts gym and feel comfortable to learn, and although there are great male and female teachers out there, it can be very intimidating for survivors. It takes tremendous strength to do something that you know will bring up old pain, but it's also a pathway to empowerment, and so I wanted to make the process easier for others by offering a stepping stone through women-only classes, and hopefully breaking down any preconceived negative ideas they may have had about training.'

DELLA O'SULLIVAN